Approach to
Clinical Endocrinology
through Selected Cases

Approach to
Clinical Endocrinology
through Selected Cases

Editors

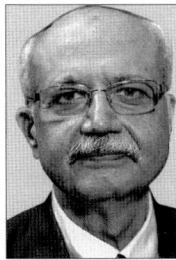

Chandar Mohan Batra
MBBS DCH MD (Internal Medicine)
DNB (Endocrinology)
Senior Consultant Endocrinologist
Department of Endocrinology
Indraprastha Apollo Hospital
New Delhi, India

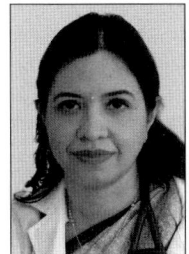

Pramila Kalra
MBBS MD (Internal Medicine)
DM (Endocrinology) MAMS FACE (USA)
FRCP (Edinburgh)
Professor and Head
Department of Endocrinology
MS Ramaiah Medical College
and Hospitals
Bengaluru, Karnataka, India

Foreword
Prasanna Kumar KM

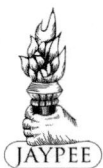

JAYPEE

JAYPEE BROTHERS MEDICAL PUBLISHERS
The Health Sciences Publisher
New Delhi | London

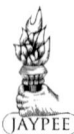 **Jaypee Brothers Medical Publishers (P) Ltd**

Headquarters
EMCA House
23/23-B, Ansari Road, Daryaganj
New Delhi 110 002, India
Landline: +91-11-23272143, +91-11-23272703
+91-11-23282021, +91-11-23245672
E-mail: jaypee@jaypeebrothers.com

Corporate Office
Jaypee Brothers Medical Publishers (P) Ltd.
4838/24, Ansari Road, Daryaganj
New Delhi 110 002, India
Phone: +91-11-43574357
Fax: +91-11-43574314
E-mail: jaypee@jaypeebrothers.com

Overseas Office
JP Medical Ltd.
83, Victoria Street, London
SW1H 0HW (UK)
Phone: +44-20 3170 8910
Fax: +44(0)20 3008 6180
E-mail: info@jpmedpub.com

Website: www.jaypeebrothers.com
Website: www.jaypeedigital.com

Inquiries for bulk sales may be solicited at: jaypee@jaypeebrothers.com

Approach to Clinical Endocrinology through Selected Cases / Chandar Mohan Batra, Pramila Kalra

First Edition: **2022**

ISBN: 978-93-89776-96-6

Printed at: Sterling Graphics Pvt. Ltd.

Dedications

The writing of his book was possible due to the efforts of a lot of people and I want to dedicate it to all of them. The Apollo Group Medical Director Dr Anupam Sibal who believed that I could write a book and sent the editor of Jaypee Brothers Medical Publishers with the proposal to me. My co-editor and co-authors collaborated with me at every step and encouraged me to continue with my efforts. My wife and daughters supported me and gave up their time with me to let me write. My parents and brothers who educated me and supported me at every step of my life. My teachers in Loyola School Jamshedpur, La Martiniere College Lucknow, King Georges Medical College Lucknow, and All India Institute of Medical Sciences (AIIMS) New Delhi trained me to become a Doctor. The three doyens of Endocrinology Professor MMS Ahuja, Professor N Kochupillai, and Professor AC Ammini at AIIMS New Delhi trained me to become an Endocrinologist and I had their blessing even after I passed out.

Dr Chandar Mohan Batra

To my parents for their support throughout my career
To my teachers who made me capable to reach this level
To my husband, daughter Sanyukta, and my brother for their constant moral support
To patients who are our best teachers.

Professor Pramila Kalra

CONTRIBUTORS

EDITORS

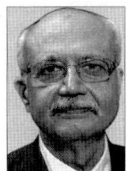

Chandar Mohan Batra
MBBS DCH MD (Internal Medicine)
DNB (Endocrinology)
Senior Consultant Endocrinologist
Department of Endocrinology
Indraprastha Apollo Hospital
New Delhi, India

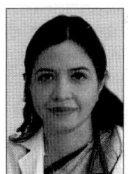

Pramila Kalra
MBBS MD (Internal Medicine) DM (Endocrinology)
MAMS FACE (USA) FRCP (Edinburgh)
Professor and Head
Department of Endocrinology
MS Ramaiah Medical College
and Hospitals
Bengaluru, Karnataka, India

CONTRIBUTING AUTHORS

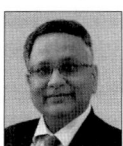

Ameet Kishore MBBS FRCS
(Glasgow) FRCS (Edinburgh)
FRCS-ORL (UK)
Senior Consultant and
Professor in ENT
Department of Neurotology
and Cochlear Implants
Indraprastha Apollo Hospital
New Delhi, India

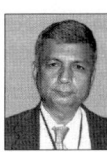

Ashok Sarin MD FRCP
Senior Consultant
Department of Nephrology
Indraprastha Apollo Hospital
New Delhi, India

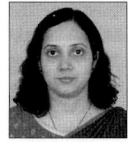

Anjana Hulse MBBS MRCPCH
(UK) MSc (Paed Sc-Endocrinology)
(Glasgow, UK)
Consultant Paediatric
Endocrinologist
Apollo Hospitals
Bengaluru, Karnataka, India

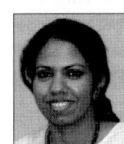

Beatrice Anne M MD DM
(Endocrinology)
Associate Professor and Head
Department of
Endocrinology
Nizam's Institute of Medical
Sciences
Hyderabad, Telangana, India

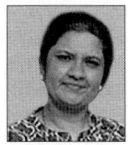

Archana Ramesh MBBS
DGO MRCOG
Consultant Obstetrics and
Gynecology
Motherhood Women and
Children's Hospital
Banashankari, Bengaluru,
Karnataka, India

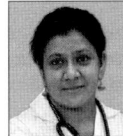

Belinda George MBBS MD
DM (Endocrinology)
Associate Professor
Department of
Endocrinology
St John's Medical College
Hospital
Bengaluru, Karnataka, India

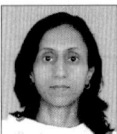

Bindu Kulshreshtha MD
DM (Endocrinology)
Professor and Head
Department of
Endocrinology
Atal Bihari Vajpayee Institute
of Medical Sciences
Dr RML Hospital
New Delhi, India

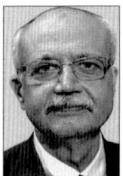

Chandar Mohan Batra
MBBS DCH MD (Internal Medicine)
DNB (Endocrinology)
Senior Consultant
Endocrinologist
Department of Endocrinology
Indraprastha Apollo
Hospitals
New Delhi, India

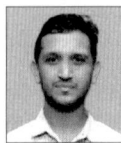

Chirag Umesh MD (Medicine)
DM (Senior Resident)
Senior Resident
Department of Endocrinology
MS Ramaiah Medical College
Bengaluru, Karnataka, India

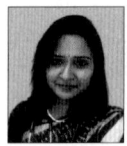

Chitra Selvan MBBS MD
(Medicine) DM (Endocrinology)
MRCP (UK) Endocrinology (sce)
Associate Professor
Department of
Endocrinology
MS Ramaiah Medical College
Bengaluru, Karnataka, India

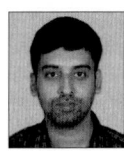

Ganesh Viswanathan MD
(Internal Medicine)
Consultant
Department of Internal
Medicine
KIMS Health
Thiruvananthapuram, Kerala,
India

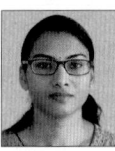

Harika Mandava MBBS
MD (Pathology)
Assistant Professor
Department of Pathology
NRI Medical College and
General Hospital
Vijayawada
Andhra Pradesh, India

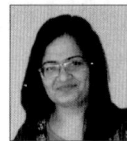

Harsha Pamnani MBBS MD
(Medicine) DNB (Endocrinology)
Consultant Endocrinologist
Department of Endocrinology
Siddhanta Red Cross
Superspeciality Hospital
Bhopal, Madhya Pradesh,
India

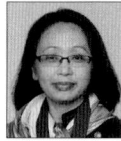

Indira Maisnam MBBS
MD DM (Endocrinology)
FRCP (Edinburgh) FACE (USA)
Consultant Endocrinologist
Department of Endocrinology
RG Kar Medical College
Kolkata, West Bengal, India

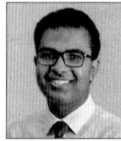

Justin Easow Sam MD DM
(Endocrinology)
Assistant Professor
Department of Endocrinology
Believers Church Medical
College, Thiruvalla
Consultant Endocrinologist
Thiruvalla Medical Mission
Hospital
Thiruvalla, Kerala, India

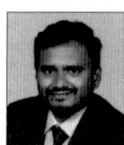

Kiran Kumar P MD
(Medicine)
2nd Year DM Resident
Department of Endocrinology
All India Institute of Medical
Sciences
New Delhi, India

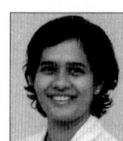

Kranti Khadilkar MBBS MD
DM (Endocrinology)
Associate Consultant
Department of Diabetes and
Endocrinology
Department of Endocrinology
Narayana Health City
Bengaluru, Karnataka, India

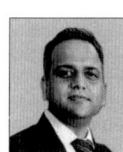

**Mohammad Asim
Siddiqui** MBBS MD (Internal
Medicine) FRCP (London)
MRCP (UK) MRCP (Endocrinology
and Diabetes)
Senior Consultant
Endocrinologist
Department of Endocrinology
Indraprastha Apollo Hospital
Jasola Vihar, New Delhi, India

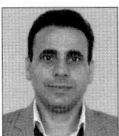

Mohd Ashraf Ganie MBBS
MD DM (Endocrinology)
Professor
Department of Endocrinology
and Metabolism
Sher-i-Kashmir Institute of
Medical Sciences
Srinagar, Jammu and
Kashmir, India

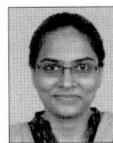

Saba Samad Memon
MBBS MD (Medicine AIIMS)
Senior Resident
Department of
Endocrinology
Seth GSMC and KEM Hospital
Mumbai, Maharashtra, India

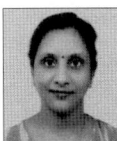

Monika Goyal MBBS MD
DNB (Endocrinology)
Assistant Professor
Department of
Endocrinology
RML Hospital
New Delhi, India

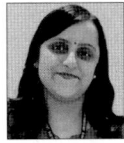

Semanti Chakarborty
MBBS MD DM (Endocrinology)
Consultant Endocrinologist
Woodlands Hospital
Kolkata, West Bengal, India

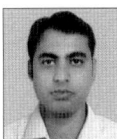

**Mukesh Kumar
Srivastava** PhD
Postdoctoral Associate
Department of Microbiology
and Immunobiology
University of Louisville
Kentucky, United States

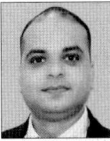

Shahid Khan PhD
Manager, Division of Genetics
Department of Pediatrics
All India Institute of Medical
Sciences
New Delhi, India

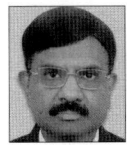

PG Sundararaman MBBS
MD DM (Endocrinology)
Senior Consultant in Medical
Endocrinology
Apollo Hospital
Billroth Hospital
Chennai, Tamil Nadu, India

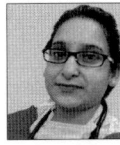

Shikha Gupta MD (Medicine)
Assistant Professor
Department of General
Medicine
Pacific Medical College
Udaipur, Rajasthan, India

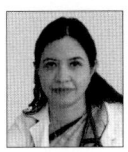

Pramila Kalra MBBS MD
(Internal Medicine)
DM (Endocrinology) MAMS FACE
(USA) FRCP (Edinburgh)
Professor and Head
Department of
Endocrinology
MS Ramaiah Medical College
and Memorial Hospital
Bengaluru, Karnataka, India

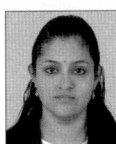

Shilpa Prabhu MBBS MD
DNB
Consultant Hematologist and
Haemato Oncologist
Narayana Multispeciality
Hospital
Bengaluru, Karnataka, India

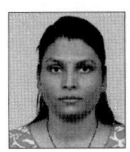

Priyanka Choudhry PHD
Consultant
Department of Indian
Pharmacopoeia Commission
Ghaziabad, Uttar Pradesh,
India

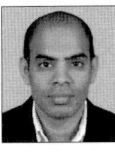

Srinivasa P Munigoti MD
(General Medicine) MRCP UK
(Diabetes and Endocrinology)
Consultant Endocrinologist
Department of Endocrinology
Fortis Hospital
Bannerghatta Road
Bengaluru, Karnataka, India

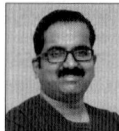

Subramaniam Kannan
MD AB (Internal Medicine and
Endocrinology) CCD ECNU
Consultant and Head
Department of Endocrinology
Narayana Hrudayalaya
Hospitals Pvt Ltd
Bengaluru, Karnataka, India

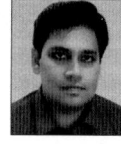

Uttio Gupta MD DM
(Endocrinology)
Consultant Endocrinologist
Department of Endocrinology
Medical Superspecialty
Hospital
Kolkata, West Bengal, India

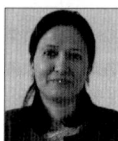

Sweety Agarwal MD DM
Consultant Endocrinology
Department of Endocrinology
Fortis Memorial Research
Institute
Gurugram, Haryana, India

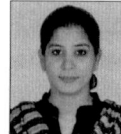

Veechika Reddy MD
(Medicine) DM Senior Resident
(Endocrinology)
Senior Resident
Department of Endocrinology
MS Ramaiah Medical College
Bengaluru, Karnataka, India

FOREWORD

After more than four decades of a clinical and academic career, I am still a clinician practicing endocrinology. We have learned a lot from our teachers and our patients, who teach us every day.

This book is a case compendium of endocrinology edited by Dr Chandar Mohan Batra and Professor Pramila Kalra. It is well written and discusses complex cases in endocrinology. Learning endocrinology or any clinical subject in medicine through cases is an innovative and exciting way to learn clinical medicine. This book is a multiauthor book written by qualified and well-experienced endocrinologists across India, both from academic and research centers in India.

I have had the opportunity to work with Dr Chandar Mohan Batra at AIIMS, New Delhi and Professor Pramila Kalra at MS Ramaiah Medical College, Bengaluru, Karnataka. They are excellent clinicians and academicians in endocrinology. Both the editors have vast experience and knowledge to edit this book and fine-tune the articles.

This book is a must for all students of endocrinology, undergraduate, postgraduate, or post-doctoral. The book has 21 chapters covering Pituitary, Thyroid, Reproductive Endocrinology, Bones, Parathyroid, Diabetes Mellitus, and Adrenal Disorders. These endocrine cases are from academic, big endocrine departments, and institutions of repute and are difficult complex cases.

This case compendium gives an insight into clinical endocrinology and how to approach an endocrine case, be it investigations, management, and follow-up. Each case is unique and will tell a story that helps a clinical endocrinologist manage such a case.

This book will help a physician, pediatrician in recognizing endocrine problems and manage or refer to a specialist. At the end of each case, there is a take home message or clinical pearls in the form of conclusions, which will help a clinician in their day-to-day management of endocrine cases.

Prasanna Kumar KM
Former Senior Professor and Head
Department of Endocrinology
MS Ramaiah Medical College and Hospital
Bengaluru, Karnataka, India
Past President—RSSDI, ESI, and Indian Thyroid Society

PREFACE

Endocrinology is a fascinating science which is easy once you have mastered the subject but for a beginner it can be complicated and difficult to understand. The best way to teach endocrinology is by presenting difficult cases. The history, examination findings, making a clinical diagnosis, investigations that are done, how the diagnosis is confirmed, and finally how the patient is treated, are the steps of a case presentation. The stepwise approach to a case makes it an interesting fascinating story that makes even the most difficult cases interesting and easy to understand. This way the reader is lead through the unraveling of a complex puzzle in the form of a story which tells them the various practical problems they will face in the management of these patients.

In this book, we have selected 21 clinical problems we face in endocrinology and tried to unravel their complexities in a simple manner.

This book will provide good learning material to practicing endocrinologists, DM and DNB students of endocrinology, internists, physicians, and general practitioners interested in endocrinology.

We are grateful to all our contributing authors, our DNB endocrinology and DM endocrinology residents for all the hard work they have put in to compile their manuscripts.

We thank our family members for the help and encouragement they gave us and finally but not the least Jaypee Brothers Medical Publishers (P) Ltd for publishing our book.

Chandar Mohan Batra
Pramila Kalra

CONTENTS

Contents

PLATE 1

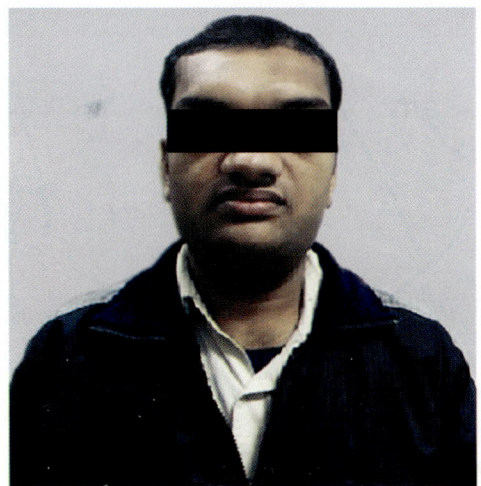

FIG. 1: Patient with facial acromegaloid features. (*Chapter 4*)

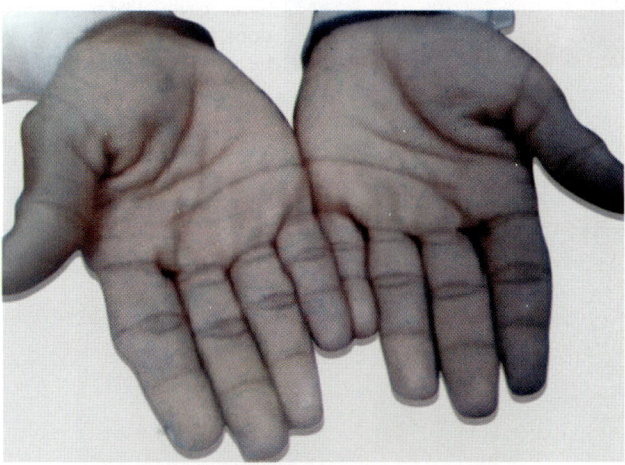

FIG. 2: Both hands showing Raynaud's phenomenon (demarcation line between discolored and normal portion). (*Chapter 4*)

PLATE 2

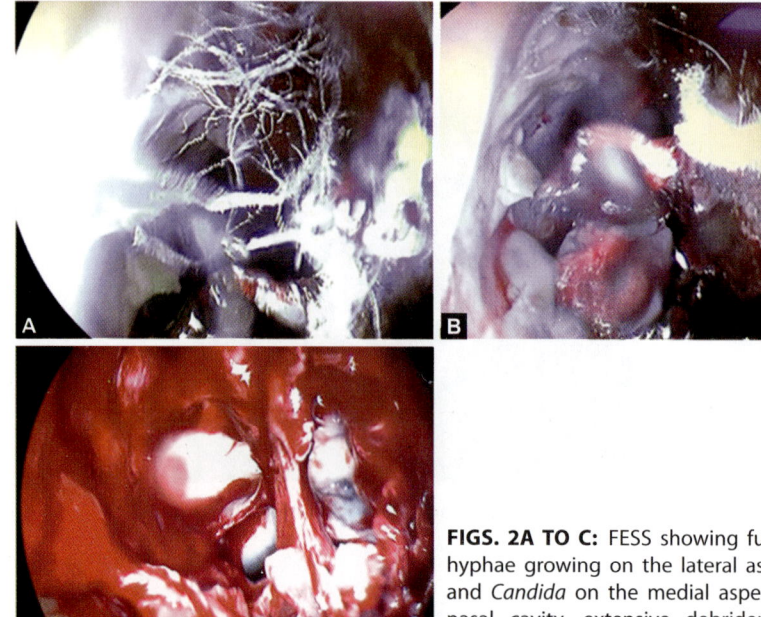

FIGS. 2A TO C: FESS showing fungal hyphae growing on the lateral aspect and *Candida* on the medial aspect of nasal cavity, extensive debridement done till normal bleeding margin can be achieved. (*Chapter 7*)

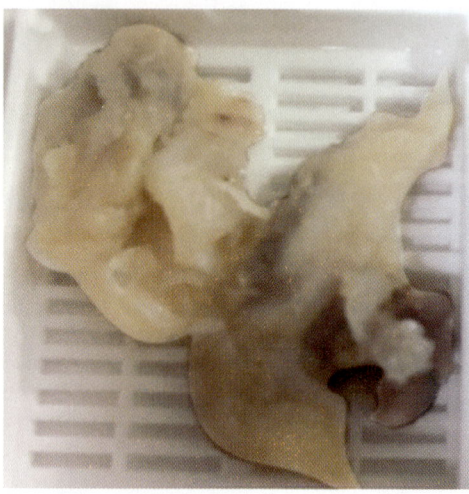

FIG. 3: Gross examination of tissue obtained on functional endoscopic sinus surgery showing dead, necrotic tissue. (*Chapter 7*)

PLATE 3

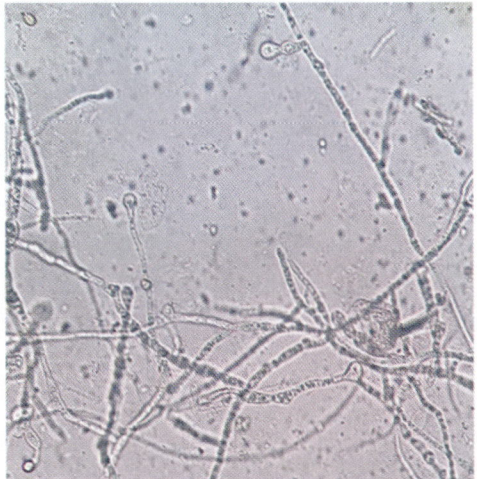

FIG. 4: KOH mount of the nasal sample showing aseptate branching fungus at right angle suggestive of mucormycosis and few budding yeast cell. (*Chapter 7*)

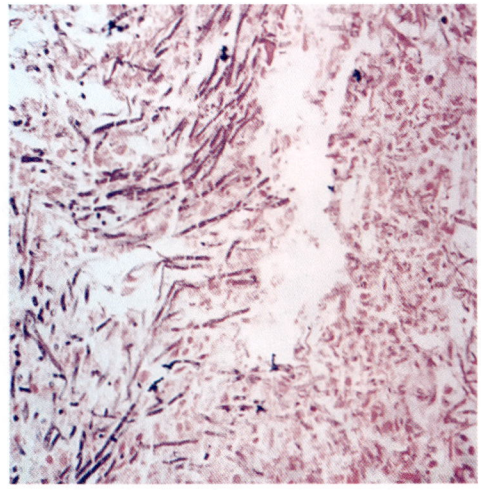

FIG. 5: Histopathological examination of biopsy tissue showing columnar epithelium, subcutaneous edema, aseptate, branching fungal growth suggestive of mucormycosis. (*Chapter 7*)

PLATE 4

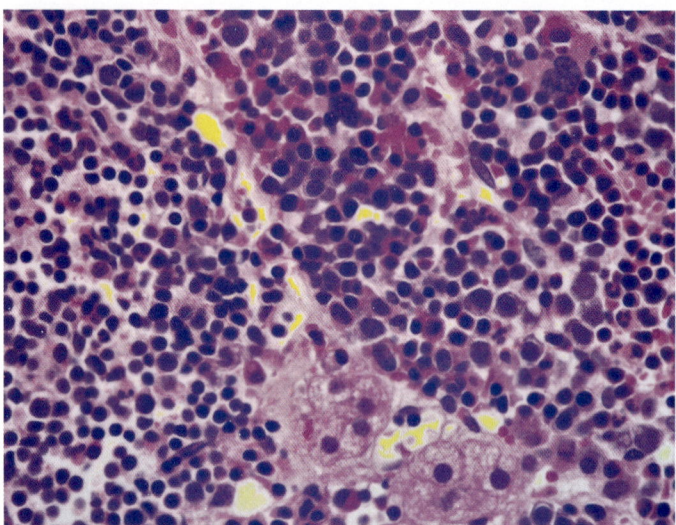

FIG. 3: Hematoxylin and eosin (H&E) stain at magnification (40×) shows adrenocortical tissue along with hematopoietic elements. It mostly shows erythroid precursors in various stages of maturation. Also seen are a few myeloid and megakaryocytic lineage cells. No adipose tissue is seen. This was consistent with a diagnosis of extramedullary hematopoiesis. (*Chapter 8*)

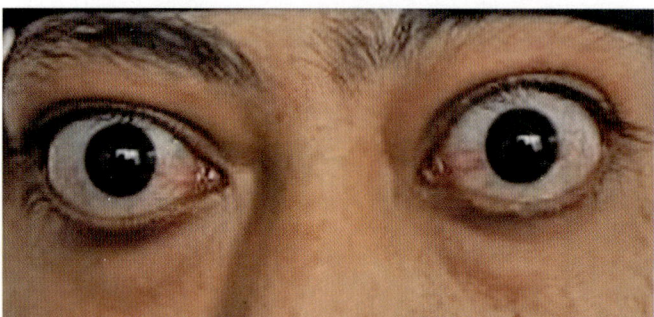

FIG. 1: Graves' orbitopathy. (*Chapter 10*)

PLATE 5

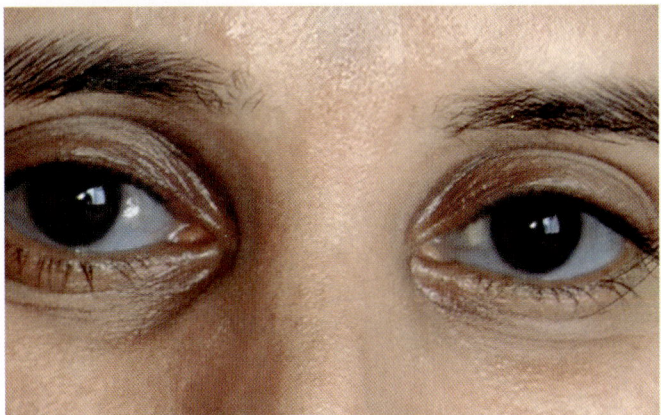

FIG. 1: Blue sclera in the mother. (*Chapter 11*)

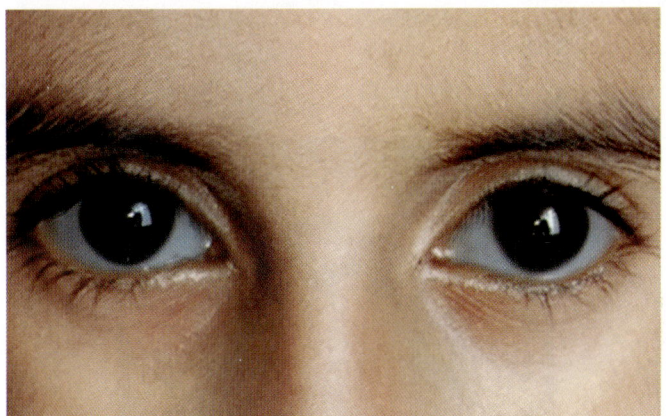

FIG. 2: Blue sclera. (*Chapter 11*)

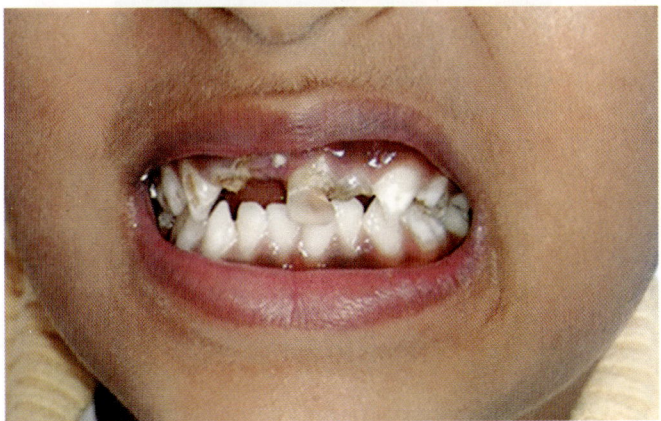

FIG. 3: Dentinogenesis imperfecta. (*Chapter 11*)

PLATE 6

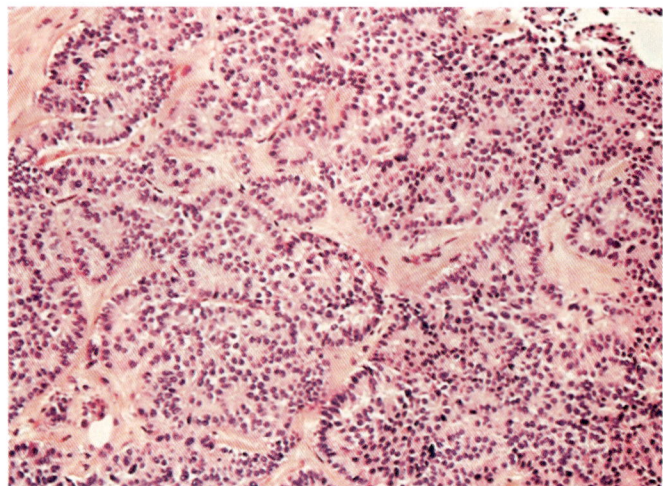

FIG. 1: Histopathology report. Well differentiated (low grade) NET of pancreas. (*Chapter 14*)

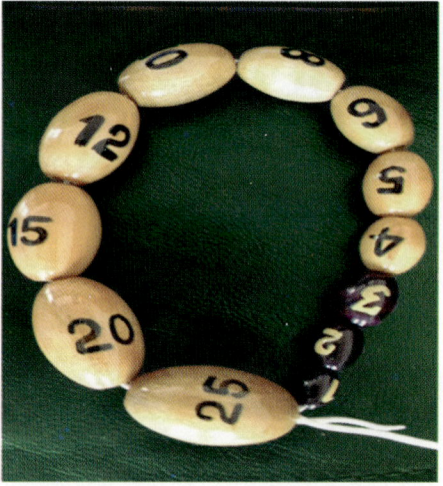

FIG. 1: Prader orchidometer. (*Chapter 16*)

Section 1: Pituitary

1

CHAPTER **Pituitary Apoplexy**

Kranti Khadilkar, Subramaniam Kannan

INTRODUCTION

Pituitary apoplexy is a clinical syndrome characterized by sudden onset of hemorrhage or infarction of the pituitary gland. It can be differentiated on the basis of acute clinical symptoms from subclinical asymptomatic pituitary apoplexy detected on routine imaging or histopathologic examination. Apoplexy usually occurs in pre-existing and often undiagnosed pituitary adenomas with an incidence of 2–7% in pituitary adenomas. The abnormal fragile vasculature in tumors and tumors outgrowing their vascular supply form the basic pathophysiology of pituitary apoplexy. Compression of the hypophyseal arteries against the diaphragma sellae due to tumor growth can also lead to ischemia and apoplexy. Hemorrhage results in increased intrasellar pressure resulting in headache and vomiting. The treatment approach can be conservative in stable cases but some cases may require urgent surgical decompression.

CASE HISTORY

Case 1

A 50-year-old gentleman presented to the emergency room (ER) with acute onset severe holocranial headache associated with projectile vomiting, dimness of vision in both eyes, and diplopia. He was hypotensive (BP 80/50 mm Hg) and hypoglycemic (capillary glucose 45 mg/dL). There was also evidence of right-sided third cranial palsy with complete right-sided ptosis and right eye mydriasis. Biochemistry in the ER showed hyponatremia (serum sodium 110 mEq/L) a random cortisol was 3 µg/dL, T4 was 3.4 ng/dL, TSH 0.05 mIU/L. MRI showed a large sellar mass extending into the right cavernous sinus with areas of acute hemorrhage in the adenoma consistent with pituitary apoplexy (**Fig. 1**). In view of hypotension, he was started on

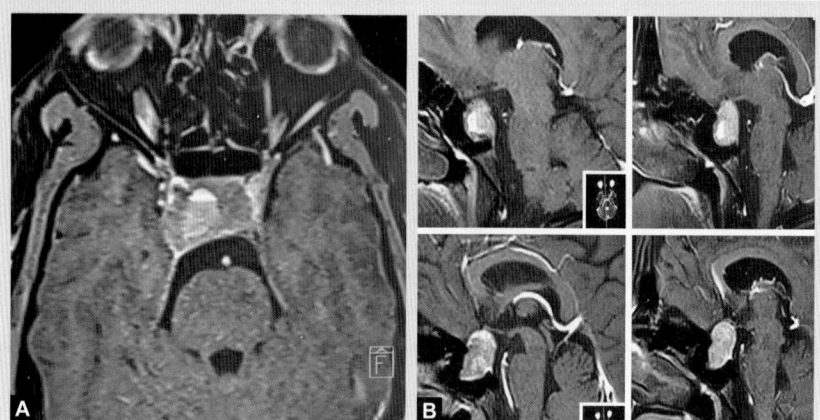

FIGS. 1A AND B: Post contrast T1W axial (A) and coronal (B) images show a pituitary macro adenoma with extension into the right cavernous sinus with evidence of hyperintense signals on T1W image indicative of acute to subacute hemorrhage.

aggressive saline infusion, intravenous hydrocortisone, and oral thyroxine and admitted in the neurosurgery ICU. Once he was hemodynamically stable, emergency surgical decompression via a transsphenoidal approach was performed. Postoperatively, patient's headache improved and on evaluation at 4 weeks in the endocrine clinic his right-sided ptosis had improved. He continues to be on hydrocortisone and levothyroxine and is on regular follow-up.

Case 2

A 25-year-old male presented with intermittent severe headaches of 2 weeks duration which was only partially relieved with analgesics. He had noticed visual blurring 2 days before presentation that was not associated with diplopia. There was no history of seizures or loss of consciousness. There were no other significant medical or surgical histories in the past. He was hemodynamically stable. Neurological examination including cranial nerves was normal except for mild blurring of optic disk on funduscopic examination. Other systemic examination did not reveal any abnormality. Magnetic resonance (MR) imaging of brain showed pituitary macroadenoma with suprasellar extension. The tumor showed internal fluid-fluid level with dependent posterior debris secondary to subacute hemorrhage (apoplexy) correlating with the history of intermittent headaches as shown in **Figure 2**. Biochemical profile revealed panhypopituitarism and mild hyponatremia. The patient was started on hydrocortisone followed by thyroxine and testosterone replacement. Serum sodium levels normalized but after a week, the headache worsened and vision deteriorated further and hence, he was subjected to transsphenoidal surgery with prompt relief of symptoms. At 3 months follow-up, he was doing well on appropriate hormonal replacement therapy.

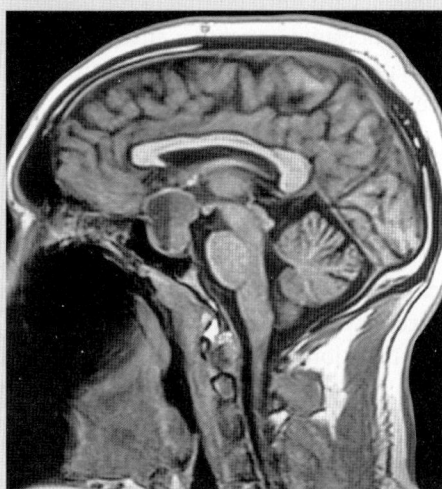

FIG. 2: MRI brain (T1W) showing pituitary macro adenoma with internal fluid-fluid level indicative of acute-subacute hemorrhage. The dependent posterior debris secondary to subacute hemorrhage (apoplexy).

DISCUSSION

Pituitary Apoplexy

Pituitary apoplexy, as the name suggests, is a clinical syndrome characterized by sudden onset hemorrhage or infarction of the pituitary gland.

Incidence of Pituitary Apoplexy

It is a rare condition with an annual incidence of 1.2 in 10,000,000. It can be differentiated on the basis of acute clinical symptoms from subclinical asymptomatic pituitary apoplexy detected on routine imaging or histo-pathologic examination. Apoplexy usually occurs in pre-existing and often undiagnosed pituitary adenomas with an incidence of 2–7% in pituitary adenomas.

Pathophysiology of Pituitary Apoplexy

The abnormal fragile vasculature in tumors and tumors outgrowing their vascular supply form the basic pathophysiology of pituitary apoplexy. Compression of the hypophyseal arteries against the diaphragma sellae due to tumor growth can also lead to ischemia and apoplexy.

Hemorrhage results in increased intrasellar pressure resulting in headache and vomiting. Extravasation to subarachnoid space causes photophobia and meningism and extravasation to cavernous sinus causes external ophthalmoplegia with third cranial nerve being the most commonly affected. Increased intracranial tension causes progressive deterioration of consciousness. Hypocortisolemia due to pituitary apoplexy causes hypotension, hyponatremia, and hypoglycemia.

Predisposing Features of Pituitary Apoplexy

Precipitating factors for pituitary apoplexy have been found in up to 40% of patients.

The precipitating factors for pituitary apoplexy are as follows:
- *Major surgery*: Coronary artery bypass grafting
- Dynamic pituitary function tests with gonadotropin-releasing hormone (GnRH), thyrotropin-releasing hormone (TRH), and corticotropin-releasing hormone (CRH)
- Anticoagulation therapy or coagulopathies
- Pregnancy
- Estrogen therapy
- Initiation or withdrawal of dopamine receptor agonist
- Radiation therapy
- Head trauma
- Acute systemic illness
- Systemic hypertension

Clinical Features of Pituitary Apoplexy

Acute onset headache holocranial or retro-orbital associated with projectile vomiting is the most common presentation of pituitary apoplexy. Neurophthalmic manifestations are present in almost two-third of the patients with visual defects and third nerve palsy being the common ones. Rare but more serious scenarios are meningism with photophobia, cerebral ischemia, and progressive loss of consciousness. Acute hypocortisolemia due to apoplexy, present in up to 70%, may result in hyponatremia and refractory hypotension. Functioning pituitary adenomas with apoplexy can, in addition, have stigmata of hormonal hypersecretion like acrogigantism, galactorrhea, and hypogonadism or cushingoid appearance.

Visual acuity, visual fields, and oculomotor nerves need to be examined in detail and progress should be charted every few hours for deterioration.

Pituitary Apoplexy Score

The Pituitary Apoplexy Score (PAS) is a simple scoring system, which can be used as an objective tool for clinical evaluation, risk stratification, and prioritization for surgery in patients with pituitary apoplexy. It is based on three parameters (visual acuity: 0, 1, and 2; visual field defect: 0, 1, and 2; and ocular paresis: 0, 1, and 2) and the Glasgow Coma Scale (GCS; 0, 2, and 4). The scoring system ranges from 0 to 10, with a higher score indicating increasing neurologic involvement.

Hormonal Studies Required in Pituitary Apoplexy

At presentation with pituitary apoplexy the majority of patients have a deficiency of one or more anterior pituitary hormones with adrenocorticotropic hormone (ACTH) being the most common (70%) along with gonadotropin deficiency (70%) followed by growth hormone (60%) and thyroid stimulating hormone (TSH) (50%). Low level of prolactin generally denotes high intrasellar pressure and poor chance of recovery of the pituitary hormonal axes.

Drawing blood samples for baseline endocrine function tests including random serum cortisol, free thyroxine (FT4), TSH, prolactin, luteinizing hormone (LH), follicle-stimulating hormone (FSH), insulin-like growth factor 1 (IGF-1), growth hormone (GH), testosterone in men and estradiol in women, serum electrolytes, clotting studies, and liver function tests (LFT) are recommended at presentation and ideally before administration of glucocorticoids.

Imaging Modalities in Pituitary Apoplexy

Magnetic resonance imaging (MRI) scanning confirms the diagnosis of pituitary apoplexy in >90% of patients and is much better than CT scan. The preoperative finding of hemorrhage or infarction on MRI scanning correlates well with the operative findings and the histopathology. The pneumonic George Washington Bridge (GWB) on T1W images helps in identifying the bleed as acute (gray), subacute (white) and black (chronic). The appearance of "OREO" cookie helps remembering the appearance on T2W images: Black (acute), white or cream (subacute), and black (chronic).

Name the Differential Diagnosis of Pituitary Apoplexy

Common medical emergencies like subarachnoid hemorrhage, migraine, meningitis, encephalitis, temporal arteritis, and cavernous sinus thrombosis are conditions which can mimic symptoms and signs of pituitary apoplexy. Hence, high degree of suspicion is required to prevent misdiagnosis.

General Supportive Care Administered in Pituitary Apoplexy

If the patient is hypotensive, resuscitation with intravenous (IV) hydration is indicated. Subsequent monitoring should include daily electrolyte measurement and fluid balance assessments and detailed neurologic and ophthalmic assessments.

Acute Management of Pituitary Apoplexy

Indications for empirical glucocorticoid treatment in patients with pituitary apoplexy are hemodynamic instability, altered consciousness level, severe visual field defects, and reduced visual acuity. In the acute setting, glucocorticoids are given most often intravenously at a stat dose of 100 mg of hydrocortisone followed by a hydrocortisone infusion at a rate of 2 mg/h or 50–100 mg intramuscular (IM) hydrocortisone every 6 hours.

The main treatment decision that is required is whether to adopt a conservative approach, or proceed to surgical decompression. The indications for a surgical decompression are a progressive reduction in visual acuity/visual fields and progressive deterioration of consciousness and neurologic assessments. Oculomotor nerve paresis in the absence of any visual field defects or reduction in visual acuity is not in itself an indication for immediate surgery. Transsphenoidal approach is usually preferred in majority of the cases; though for giant pituitary adenomas a transcranial approach may be required. The improvement usually starts immediately postoperatively and continues for several weeks. Visual recovery is less likely in patients presenting with monocular or binocular blindness, and early surgical decompression again is more likely to achieve best visual outcomes.

Retrospective studies have not shown any statistically significant differences in the endocrine outcomes between patients managed medically versus those managed surgically. However, majority of these uncontrolled studies have a selection bias.

Postoperative management of patients after surgery for pituitary apoplexy is similar to other elective pituitary surgeries. Anterior pituitary function needs to be tested postoperatively: 9 AM cortisol is usually checked on day 3 postoperatively along with thyroid function (FT4 and TSH). If there is cortisol deficiency prior to the surgical intervention, then hydrocortisone is usually continued and changed to maintenance dose when the patient is stable, with further assessment of cortisol 4–8 weeks later. In up to 50% of patients, partial or complete recovery of pituitary function is observed after the acute event.

Long-term Prognosis and Follow-up in Cases of Pituitary Apoplexy

Up to 80% of patients with pituitary apoplexy require one or more pituitary hormone replacement in the long term with most common being glucocorticoid replacement followed by thyroid and sex steroids. Initial endocrine assessment should be done at 4–8 weeks after the acute episode followed by annual assessment. MRI Imaging should be repeated at 3–6 months after the episode followed by annual MRI imaging for 5 years. Progressive regrowth as well as recurrent apoplexy can occur in both surgically and conservatively managed patients, hence the importance of annual follow-up imaging and endocrine assessment.

CONCLUSION

Pituitary apoplexy is an endocrine emergency requiring a high index of suspicion for its timely diagnosis and appropriate management. Acute glucocorticoid replacement is required in hemodynamically unstable patients whereas urgent neurosurgical decompression is indicated in progressive deterioration of consciousness and neuro-ophthalmic status. Effective treatment requires experienced endocrine and neurosurgical services.

SUGGESTED READINGS

1. Barkhoudarian G, Kelly DF. Pituitary Apoplexy. Neurosurg Clin N Am. 2019;30(4):457-63.
2. Muthukumar N. Pituitary Apoplexy: A Comprehensive Review. Neurol India. 2020;68 (Supplement):S72-S78.
3. Rajasekaran S, Vanderpump M, Baldeweg S, et al. UK guidelines for the management of pituitary apoplexy. Clin Endocrinol (Oxf). 2011;74(1):9-20.
4. Reddy NL, Rajasekaran S, Han TS, et al. An objective scoring tool in the management of patients with pituitary apoplexy. Clin Endocrinol (Oxf). 2011;75(5):723.
5. Sibal L, Ball SG, Connolly V, et al. Pituitary apoplexy: a review of clinical presentation, management and outcome in 45 cases. Pituitary. 2004;7(3):157-63.

2

CHAPTER

Approach to Cerebral Salt Wasting

Ganesh Viswanathan, Belinda George

INTRODUCTION

Cerebral salt wasting (CSW) is an uncommon cause of hyponatremia, a hydroelectrolytic disorder with serum level of sodium <135 mEq/L. Hyponatremia presents mild-to-severe symptoms such as confusion, nausea, vomiting, lethargy, fatigue, hiccups, seizures, and coma due to several factors such as adrenal disorders, syndrome of inappropriate antidiuretic hormone (SIADH), or certain medications such as diuretics, antidepressants, or pain medications. In critical care setting, the rate of hyponatremia traumatic subarachnoid hemorrhage (SAH) is as high as 30%. Here, we report a case of 31-year-old with head injury who developed CSW due to SAH.

CASE 1

A 31-year-old male was admitted to intensive care unit (ICU) following a road traffic accident with history suggestive of head injury. He was in altered sensorium with a Glasgow Coma Scale (GCS) of 6/15 and had an episode of generalized tonic-clonic seizures on the way to the hospital. His CT of the brain revealed a large SAH with intraventricular extension. He was managed in the neurosurgical ICU and was extubated after 6 days once his clinical condition improved.

However, his sensorium worsened again and he was detected to have hyponatremia with serum sodium of 122 mEq/L and serum osmolality of 266 mOsm/kg.

---

1. **What is hyponatremia and how often does it occur in the critical care setting?**

    Hyponatremia is defined as a serum level of sodium <135 mEq/L. The common symptoms associated with hyponatremia are confusion, lethargy, fatigue, hiccoughs, seizures, and coma. It is especially common in a critical care setting with traumatic SAH where rates as high as 30% has been reported.

2. Why is hyponatremia very common in critically ill and neurosurgical patients?

The complex mechanism involved in maintaining sodium and water balance is mainly carried out by the central nervous system and the kidneys. Sodium is predominantly regulated by the renin–angiotensin–aldosterone system (RAAS) and water metabolism is predominantly regulated by antidiuretic hormone (ADH) or arginine vasopressin (AVP) secreted from the hypothalamus. Many disease states can affect these processes, particularly the ADH secretion; hence, it is common to encounter abnormalities of sodium and water homeostasis in critically ill patients, especially in those with central nervous system involvement.

3. What is osmolality?

Osmolality is defined as the concentration of a solution expressed in osmoles of solute particles per kilogram of the solvent irrespective of its (solute's) size or electrical charge. In the serum, osmolality refers to the number of dissolved particles per kilogram of water. When the number of solute particles is less in proportion to the number of units of water, it will become hypo-osmolar solution (less concentration of solute with more water); when the number of solute particles is more in proportion to the number of units of water, it will become a hyperosmolar solution (high concentration of solute with less water).

4. What is the difference between osmolality, osmolarity, and tonicity?

Osmolality and osmolarity—both these terms refer to measurement of osmotic activity of a given solution. These measurements may be expressed as osmoles or milliosmoles. Osmosis refers to a process in which molecules in a solvent passes through a semipermeable membrane from one compartment (usually higher in solutes) to another compartment (lower number of solutes) based on the concentration gradient of solutes it contains (**Box 1**).

BOX 1 | **Back to chemistry for some basic definitions.**

- Mole—the amount of a given substance that contains molecules equal to the number called as Avogadro's number
- Avogadro's number—6.022×1023; the number of molecules contained in one mole of a substance
- Molality—number of moles of solute per kilogram of solvent
- Molarity—number of moles of solute per liter of solution
- Osmole—amount of substance that contains exact number of particles (Avogadro's number) that will depress the freezing point of the solvent by 1.86°C
- Osmolality—number of osmoles of solute per kilogram of solvent
- Osmolarity—number of osmoles of solute per liter of solution

Osmolarity refers to the number of milliosmoles present in 1 L of solution (mOsm/L)—refers to concentration of a solution. The plasma osmolarity in humans ranges between 270 and 300 mOsm/L.

Osmolality refers to the number of milliosmoles per kilogram of the solvent—refers to concentration of particles dissolved in the fluid. This is the measurement used clinically when we evaluate disorders of water and sodium homeostasis. The serum osmolality in humans ranges between 280 and 295 mOsm/kg.

Tonicity is another term used frequently in medical parlance and loosely refers to osmolality of a solution in comparison with plasma (i.e., hypotonic, isotonic, or hypertonic). However, the accurate definition of tonicity refers to the effective osmolality of a solution and is approximately equal to the sum of solute particles which are not freely permeable across the cell membrane and, hence, has the ability to exert an osmotic pressure across the membrane based on its concentration gradient. Any solute that is freely permeable across the cell membrane becomes an ineffective osmole (e.g., urea), as the solute itself will move across the membrane to maintain equilibrium.

In clinical situations, it is the effective osmolality that is important rather than the measured osmolality that is assessed in the laboratory using the freezing point depression method. As sodium is the largest contributor to osmolality in serum, osmolality and sodium concentrations usually parallel each other. Hyponatremia is likely to be associated with hypo-osmolar serum and hypernatremia is associated with hyperosmolar serum.

5. How is osmolality measured in the laboratory?

The laboratory measurement of osmolality of fluids utilizes their colligative properties rather than direct measurement of their osmotic pressure. The commonly used property is the ability of a fluid to depress the freezing point of water. Solute-free pure water freezes at 0°C. If one osmole of any solute (or a combination of solutes) is added to water, it will depress the freezing point of one kilogram of water by 1.86°C. This property is utilized to measure osmolality of body fluids by measuring the depression in freezing point to assess the number of osmoles present. The freezing point of serum is approximately –0.521°C, which corresponds to an osmolality of 0.280 Osm/kg or 280 mOsm/kg.

6. How is osmolality calculated? What are the main solutes affecting osmolality?

The formula for calculating serum osmolality is as follows:

$$\text{Serum osmolality} = 2 \times (Na^+ + K^+) + \text{Blood urea nitrogen}/2.8 + \text{Glucose}/18$$

Blood urea nitrogen (in mg/dL)
Plasma glucose (in mg/dL)
Sodium and potassium (in mEq/L)

The formula takes the main solutes dissolved in plasma into consideration while calculating the osmolality value. However, both urea and glucose are ineffective osmoles as they can freely pass through the cell membranes from the intracellular fluid (ICF) compartment to the extracellular fluid (ECF) compartment and vice versa. This makes sodium the most effective osmole in circulation. Glucose could become an effective osmole in the absence or deficiency of insulin (e.g., hyperosmolar hyperglycemic syndrome).

7. What are the factors involved in physiological regulation of water metabolism?

Vasopressin is the main hormone involved in the regulation of water homeostasis and, thereby, contributes to maintaining serum osmolality in the normal range. In normal subjects, the serum osmolality ranges from 280 to 295 mOsm/kg; however, in any given individual, it is maintained within a much narrower range. The ability to maintain this narrow range is dependent on the sensitive response of plasma vasopressin to changes in serum osmolality and the sensitive response of the urine osmolality and urine volume to the change in vasopressin levels.

Vasopressin is a nonapeptide, which is stored and secreted from the posterior pituitary. It is synthesized in the magnocellular neurons of the paraventricular and supraoptic hypothalamic nuclei and then transported to the distal axons located in the posterior pituitary. Basal vasopressin levels in humans ranges from 0.5 to 2 pg/mL. An increase or decrease in plasma osmolality (even as little as 1%) has the ability to cause a rapid increase or decrease in vasopressin secretion from the posterior pituitary. The secreted vasopressin is also quickly metabolized (half-life ~15 min) permitting rapid changes in circulating vasopressin levels. In the kidney, vasopressin acts in the collecting duct by increasing aquaporin channel expression and facilitating water extraction from the urine.

The changes in blood volume and blood pressure required to stimulate vasopressin are much higher (~10–15%); these are maintained predominantly via the RAAS. When the effective osmotic pressure of the plasma rises, vasopressin secretion is increased and the thirst mechanism is stimulated. Water is retained in the body, diluting the hypertonic plasma, and water intake is increased. Conversely, when the plasma becomes hypotonic, vasopressin secretion is decreased and "solute-free water" (water in excess of solute) is excreted.

8. What are the physiological mechanisms involved in sodium metabolism?

The main regulator of sodium homeostasis and maintenance of blood volume and systemic vascular resistance is the RAAS. Renin, which is released from the kidneys, stimulates formation of angiotensin II, which, in turn, stimulates aldosterone secretion from the adrenal cortex. Angiotensin II acts via several mechanisms to improve blood volume and pressure: (i) constriction of blood vessels and increase in peripheral vascular resistance, (ii) increased reabsorption of sodium and water from renal tubules, (iii) increased secretion of aldosterone, (iv) increased secretion of vasopressin, (v) increased sensation of thirst, and (vi) enhances sympathetic adrenergic function. Aldosterone additionally acts on the epithelial sodium channels located in the distal nephrons to enhance sodium reabsorption. The RAAS is under the local regulation within the kidney based on afferent arteriolar pressure (juxtaglomerular apparatus) and the solute density reaching the distal tubule (macula densa).

Sodium and free water excretion from the kidney is also influenced by other hormones such as tetraiodothyronine, cortisol, and growth hormone. Hence, it is important to exclude thyroid dysfunction and hypoadrenalism while evaluating for hyponatremia, especially, if euvolemic.

9. What are the main etiologies for hyponatremia encountered in the neurointensive care unit?

The most common diagnosis in a patient with an intracranial pathology along with hyponatremia is syndrome of inappropriate antidiuresis (SIAD). However, it is important to exclude other rare causes such as pituitary insufficiency and CSW syndrome, as these causes may also be seen in the setting of head injury. Accurate diagnosis of the etiology of hyponatremia is imperative, as the therapeutic considerations differ significantly based on the diagnosis. A delay in the institution of appropriate management may lead to worsening clinical condition and even death.

10. What is cerebral salt wasting? How was it described first?

Cerebral salt wasting is a disorder of water and sodium homeostasis with inappropriate urinary salt losses in the setting of reduced effective arterial blood volume. The initial reports were from neurosurgical patients with cerebral disease and normal renal function; hence, the etiology of renal loss was attributed to the brain pathology.

The very first descriptions of CSW were by Peters et al. in 1950 from Yale hospital. Yale hospital was one of the first medical centers to acquire the flame photometer, a medical device that could determine sodium concentrations in body fluids. Peters described three patients treated in Yale hospital for central nervous system pathologies and hyponatremia. All three patients had persistent urinary sodium loss, despite hyponatremia and clinical signs of dehydration. SIAD had not been then described in literature.

A landmark paper by Schwartz et al. in 1957 describing SIADH and its clinical features suggested that increased levels of vasopressin or ADH lead to hyponatremia and natriuresis associated with water retention and weight gain. Though the patients described in SIADH series were those with bronchogenic carcinoma, the authors noticed the similarities between theirs and the earlier series and mentioned that increased ADH could be the mechanism for hyponatremia in those with nervous system disease as well. There was a subsequent publication from the Yale group, which attributed the hyponatremia in neurological disease to be mediated by increased ADH.

The description of SIADH changed the consensus on the concept of CSW syndrome and it was now considered to be either nonexistent or a part or spectrum of SIADH itself. The term CSW disappeared from literature; only three articles can be found on MEDLINE search on CSW dated before 1981. A resurgence of CSW occurred from 1981 onward when a paper published by Nelson et al. described hyponatremia in neurosurgical patients who were found to have contracted blood volumes (measured isotopically) as opposed to expanded blood volume that was expected in SIADH. He attributed the cause for hyponatremia to CSW and it has been recognized as a separate entity since then.

11. How common is CSW in patients presenting with neurological disease and hyponatremia?

A study done using retrospective data collection from medical records of patients with SAH and hyponatremia found that the diagnosis was SIADH in 69% of patients and CSW was thought to contribute to hyponatremia in only 6.5% of patients. Though CSW is a relatively uncommon cause for hyponatremia (~10 times less common than SIADH), it is important to consider it as a differential and make an accurate diagnosis.

12. What are the similarities between SIAD and CSW? Why is it important to make the differentiation in your diagnosis?

The clinical setting in which we are likely to encounter these are similar. It includes head trauma, intracranial hemorrhage, intracranial neoplasms, malignancy, infectious meningitis, and following neurosurgical procedures and surgery. Both conditions will have hyponatremia with increased urinary loss of sodium. The theoretical difference is that one has an expanded or normal blood volume, whereas, in CSW, there is relative reduction in effective arterial blood volume.

Restriction of water or fluid intake will help in the case of SIADH; however, volume contraction can worsen and hyponatremia may become severe, if the same is attempted on a patient with CSW. As the treatment modalities are opposite for these two conditions, it is crucial for the treating team to arrive at an accurate diagnosis.

> ### Case 1 Cont'd...
>
> His sensorium worsened and he was detected to have hyponatremia with serum sodium of 122 mEq/L and serum osmolality of 266 mOsm/kg. His intake in the last 24 hours was 4,200 mL and a urine output of 3,500 mL. The urinary osmolality was 534 mOsmol/kg and the urinary sodium was 74 mEq/L.

13. What is the likely diagnosis? What additional information is needed to make an informed decision?

As the most common etiology for hyponatremia in this clinical setting is SIAD, it would be right to consider it as the first diagnosis. However, it is important to evaluate the patient's volume status before doing so (**Box 2**).

> ### Case 1 Cont'd...
>
> The patient appeared euvolemic clinically with a heart rate of 88 beats/min, blood pressure of 120/80 mm Hg, no postural drop, and no edema or ascites. Laboratory evaluation revealed normal thyroid and adrenal functions.
>
> A diagnosis of SIAD was made and fluid restriction to 1 L/day was started. However, the sodium levels worsened and patient's clinical situation deteriorated.

14. Was the diagnosis of SIAD wrong?

Based on the diagnostic criteria for the diagnosis of SIAD, a low serum osmolality in the presence of clinical euvolemia and renal salt wasting as mentioned below suggests the underlying etiology to be SIAD.

BOX 2	Diagnostic criteria for syndrome of inappropriate antidiuresis (SIAD).

Essential features:
- Effective serum osmolality <275 mOsm/kg
- Urine osmolality >100 mOsm/kg during hypotonicity
- Clinical euvolemia
- Urine sodium concentration >30 mmol/L with normal dietary salt intake
- Normal adrenal, thyroid, pituitary, and renal function
- No recent use of diuretic agents

Supplemental features:
- Serum uric acid <0.24 mmol/L (<4 mg/dL)
- Serum urea <3.6 mmol/L (<21.6 mg/dL)
- Failure to correct hyponatremia after 0.9% saline infusion
- Fractional sodium excretion >0.5%
- Fractional urea excretion >55%
- Fractional uric acid excretion >12%
- Correction of hyponatremia through fluid restriction

However, as restriction of fluids lead to worsening of hyponatremia, the diagnosis needs to be reconsidered. The possibility that both disorders might coexist should also be considered.

15. What are the proposed mechanisms of CSW?

The exact mechanism by which central nervous system disease causes CSW is poorly understood. The primary pathology is considered to be natriuresis leading to hypovolemia and sodium depletion in the absence of a known triggering factor that promotes renal salt wasting. Several natriuretic factors have been proposed to play a role in the pathogenesis of CSW including atrial natriuretic peptide (ANP), brain natriuretic peptide (BNP), C-type natriuretic peptide (CNP), and dendroaspis natriuretic peptide (DNP). Among them, BNP is considered to be the most likely candidate, as it is secreted and released from the brain, and is likely to be altered in intracranial disease.

These factors increase urinary excretion of sodium via a direct inhibitory effect on the intramedullary collecting duct sodium absorption and also by directly inhibiting renal tubular sodium reabsorption. They may act directly on juxtaglomerular apparatus to decrease renin release leading to lower aldosterone concentrations. Additionally, they have direct inhibitory effect on aldosterone release from adrenals. This suppression of RAAS leads to renal salt wasting. These natriuretic peptides are capable of increasing renal sodium excretion independent of potassium depletion.

Following an intracranial insult, the natriuretic peptides may increase from increased surges of sympathetic outflow leading to atrial stretch or increased ventricular load. Direct damage to brain structures housing BNP may lead to unregulated release of BNP into circulation during an SAH or other intracranial insults. The hypothalamus, which is the structure responsible for storage and release of ANP and BNP, may generate and secrete these natriuretic peptides in response to rising intracranial pressures as a defense mechanism to protect the neurons from permanent damage.

Several studies have attempted to correlate these natriuretic factors and occurrence of CSW; however, none of the studies have shown that they are unequivocally elevated in all brain injury patients developing CSW. Hence, additional mechanisms either involving a combination of factors or driven by an entirely novel endogenous compound that is yet unidentified cannot be ruled out.

Another commonly proposed theory is that of disrupted neural inputs to the kidney, which leads to decreased sodium reabsorption from the proximal tubule. This eventually leads to an increased delivery of sodium to the distal tubule, increased sodium excretion, and a decrease in effective arterial blood volume (EABV); the decrease in EABV, in turn, activates the baroreceptors and stimulates AVP release (**Flowchart 1**).

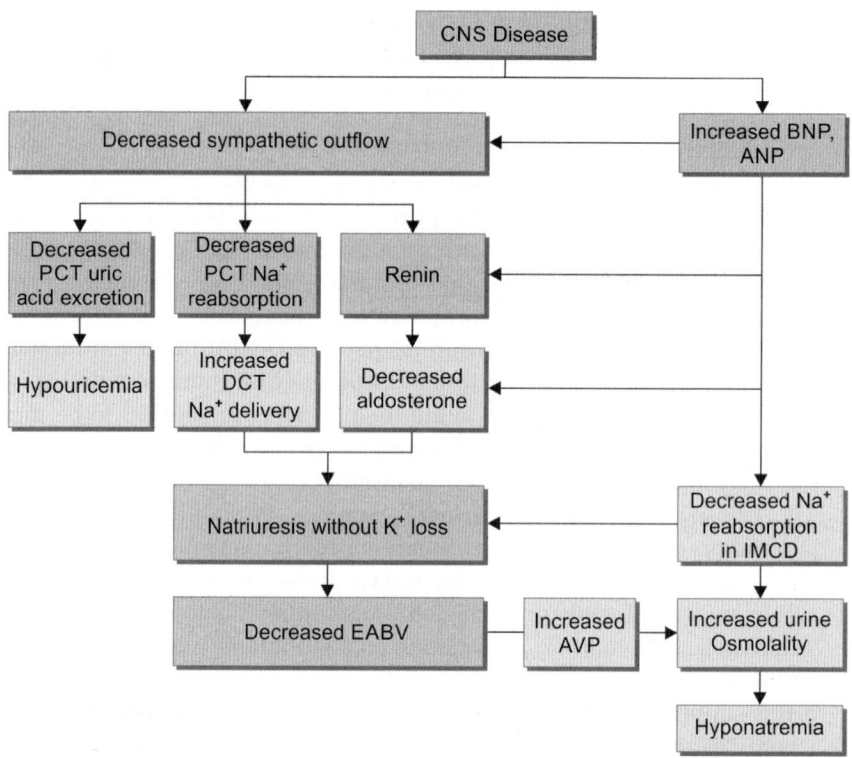

(ANP: atrial natriuretic peptide; AVP: arginine vasopressin; BNP: brain natriuretic peptide; CNS: central nervous system; CSW: cerebral salt wasting; DCT: distal convoluted tubule; EABV: effective arterial blood volume; IMCD: inner medullary collecting duct; PCT: proximal convoluted tubule)

FLOWCHART 1: Proposed mechanisms for CSW.

16. What are the clinical clues and investigations that could help us to differentiate between CSW and SIAD?

The fundamental difference between CSW and SIAD is that in CSW, there is a reduction in EABV and in SIAD, the EABV is either normal or slightly expanded. Accurate assessment of intravascular volume needs isotope studies and is impractical at the bedside. At times, the clinical picture may be very similar in both patients, making it difficult to differentiate the two. However, hyponatremia with reduced serum osmolality and increased natriuresis in the presence of volume contraction should point toward CSW. Symptoms and signs of dehydration, low central venous pressure, and hemoconcentration (raised hematocrit, elevated blood urea and creatinine, increased serum albumin, and bicarbonate levels) are diagnostic clues that favor CSW. Serum uric acid levels tend to be reduced in both conditions in the initial phase; however, uric acid excretion has been suggested as a way of differentiating the two.

TABLE 1: Differentiating CSW from SIAD.

Symptoms	CSW	SIAD
EABV	Decreased	Normal/Increased
Dehydration	Present	Absent
Weight	Decreased	Normal/Increased
Plasma albumin/Protein ratio	Increased	Normal
Central venous pressure	Decreased	Increased/Normal
Osmolality	Decreased	Decreased
Hematocrit	Increased	Decreased/Normal
Serum urea nitrogen/Creatinine ratio	Increased	Normal
Serum K^+ concentration	Increased/Normal	Decreased/Normal
Plasma uric acid	Decreased	Decreased
Fractional excretion of uric acid (initial)	High	High
Fractional excretion of uric acid (after correction)	High	Normal
Treatment	Fluids and/or Mineralocorticoids	Restriction of fluids

(CSW: cerebral salt wasting; EABV: effective arterial blood volume; SIAD: syndrome of inappropriate antidiuresis)

Uric acid is normally reabsorbed from the proximal tubule along with sodium. In patients with SIAD, due to expanded ECF volume, sodium reabsorption in the PCT is reduced and, hence, uric acid excretion is also increased leading to low uric acid levels in the serum. The stimulation of V1 receptors by ADH is also known to increase uric acid excretion in the renal tubules. The exact mechanism of decreased uric acid in CSW has not been identified yet, but is thought to occur as a part of solute diuresis with impaired uric acid absorption in the proximal tubules. The main difference between the two conditions is that in SIAD, correction of hyponatremia leads to normalization of serum uric acid level and fractional excretion of uric acid. However, in CSW, the abnormalities persist even after correction of sodium. **Table 1** summarizes the key differences between SIAD and CSW.

17. Mention some dynamic tests that have been suggested to differentiate between CSW and SIAD.

Some diagnostic tests have been proposed to discriminate between SIAD and CSW.

- Furosemide infusion test—infusion of 20 mg of furosemide would lead to increase in sodium levels in SIAD but worsening in CSW. Care should be taken to do this provocative test under continuous monitoring.

  Safety and reproducibility of these have not been validated; hence, they are not advised in routine clinical practice.

18. What is the fundamental difference in the management of CSW and SIAD?

The treatment of choice for SIAD is free water restriction; an increase in fluid intake typically worsens the hyponatremia associated with SIAD. On the contrary, hyponatremia associated with CSW requires adequate replacement with isotonic or hypertonic saline, as it is a volume-depleted state with renal salt wasting.

If the patient is symptomatic and the hyponatremia is severe, one could commence treatment with hypertonic saline, irrespective of the diagnosis. However, it is imperative to reassess the situation frequently and accurately to decide the further course of management (fluid restriction vs. liberal replacement).

19. What other therapeutic options are available for CSW?

A combination of urea and saline has been tried in patients with intracranial disease where the diagnosis is unclear. Urea acts as a mild osmotic diuretic, which depresses urinary sodium excretion and NaCl acts to reduce the sodium deficit. It is necessary to guard against rapid correction of hyponatremia in order to avoid osmotic demyelination syndrome.

Fludrocortisone has been used in isolated cases in doses of 0.05–0.1 mg twice daily with effective results. It directly acts on the renal tubule to enhance sodium reabsorption. Adverse effects such as hypokalemia, pulmonary edema, and hypertension may occur, if used for prolonged duration. It should only be used as a second line of treatment in cases where fluid management and salt replacement fail.

The new class of drugs called vaptans (vasopressin antagonists) should not be used in CSW, as they are relatively contraindicated in hypovolemic hyponatremia.

20. How should one approach hyponatremia?

One should approach to hyponatremia as described in **Flowchart 2**.

DISCUSSION

Hyponatremia is an electrolyte abnormality frequently observed in patients with aneurysmal SAH. In any clinical setting, the diagnosis should be based on the history (including drug history) and examination of cardiac, endocrine, pulmonary, and renal function with special attention to neurological examination. Complete hormone profile, serum and urine biochemical parameters, and patient's volume status should be evaluated and other rare causes such as pituitary insufficiency, CSW syndrome, thyroid dysfunction, and hypoadrenalism should be excluded, especially if hyponatremia is euvolemic. For analysis of etiology of hyponatremia, determination of serum and urine osmolarity should also be done. Accurate diagnosis of the etiology of hyponatremia is imperative, as the therapeutic

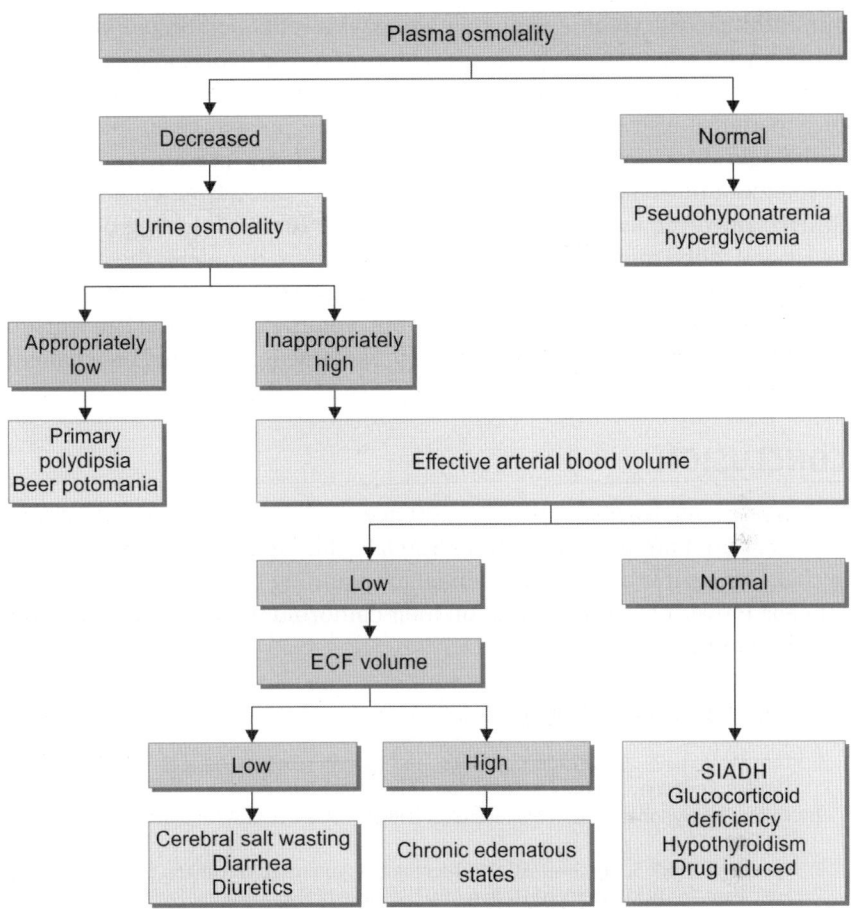

(ECF: extracellular fluid; SIADH: syndrome of inappropriate antidiuretic hormone)

FLOWCHART 2: Approach to hyponatremia.

considerations differ significantly based on the diagnosis. Early diagnosis is also essential to undermine the associated complications. Any delay in the institution of appropriate management may lead to worsening of clinical condition and even death. Both SIADH and CSW syndrome are reported to be a major cause of hyponatremia. While the treatment of choice for SIADH is free water restriction, an increase in fluid intake typically worsens the hyponatremia associated with SIADH. On the contrary, CSW results in sodium losses without any change in volume expansion. This pathogenesis of CSW can be implicated to sympathetic innervation to the kidney. In the absence of adrenal insufficiency, renal dysfunction, or inappropriate volume expansion, CSW should be considered in any at-risk patient with abnormal sodium handling. In severe conditions, CSW results in high urine sodium concentration and high urine output that leads to high serum urea. The first line of management in such cases should be correction of hyponatremia and intravascular volume depletion along with reduction of loss of urinary sodium with adequate replacement with isotonic or hypertonic saline. But, close monitoring is essential to prevent volume overload that might lead to hypertension and pulmonary edema. In the present case, intracranial pathology along with low serum osmolality in the presence of clinical euvolemia and renal salt wasting suggested the underlying etiology to be SIADH. However, as restriction of fluids lead to further lowering of sodium levels and worsening of patient's clinical condition, therefore, the diagnosis was reconsidered. This can be justified by the fact that restriction of water or fluid intake helps in cases of SIADH; but, volume contraction can worsen and hyponatremia may become severe, if the same is attempted on a patient with CSW.

CONCLUSION

The case report highlights the importance of distinguishing the common cause of hyponatremia—CSW from SIADH. Although the precise diagnosis is challenging, it is absolutely essential for planning personalized treatment for each individual patient based on their comorbidities and type and cause of hyponatremia.

SUGGESTED READINGS

1. Loh JA, Verbalis JG. Disorders of Water and Salt Metabolism Associated with Pituitary Disease. Endocrinol Metab Clin North Am. 2008;37:213-34.
2. Palmer BF. Hyponatremia in neurosurgical patient: SIADH vs CSW. Nephrol Dial Transplant. 2000;15:262-8.
3. Fenske W, Störk S, Koschker AC, Blechschmidt A, Lorenz D, Wortmann S, et al. Value of Fractional Uric Acid Excretion in Differential Diagnosis of Hyponatremic Patients on Diuretics. J Clin Endocrinol Metab. 2008;93:2991-7.
4. Betjes MGH. Hyponatremia in acute brain disease: the cerebral salt wasting syndrome. Eur J Intern Med. 2002;13:9-14.

3

CHAPTER **Sheehan's Syndrome**

Indira Maisnam

INTRODUCTION

Sheehan's syndrome is postpartum pituitary failure due to pituitary infarction following massive postpartum hemorrhage (PPH). It is not an uncommon cause of hypopituitarism in certain regions of the world. A chronic and progressive condition, diagnosis of Sheehan's is often delayed because of nonspecific symptoms and lack of awareness, thereby increasing disease-associated morbidity and mortality. Timely diagnosis and replacement of deficient hormone improves quality of life.

CASE HISTORY

Case 1

A 42-year-old lady was brought to the emergency department with acute onset confusion and drowsiness. She had been unwell for the past 1 week due to fever, cough and expectoration, and had taken some over-the-counter medication but her symptoms persisted.

On examination, she was drowsy with a Glasgow Coma Scale (GCS) of 8/15 and a temperature of 102°F. Her pulse was 68/min and regular; BP was 86/60 mm Hg. She was anemic with poor nutrition; had fine wrinkling around the eyes and the mouth; and had sparse axillary and pubic hair with breast atrophy. On chest auscultation, there were crepitations in the right infra-axillary region. There was no neck rigidity and plantar reflex was bilaterally nonresponsive.

Emergency reports showed neutrophilic leukocytosis and serum sodium of 115 mg/dL. Urine osmolality and urinary sodium were high at 370 mOsmol/kg and 44 mEq/L. Random capillary blood glucose was 55 mg/dL. Chest X-ray showed a pneumonic consolidation in the right lower lobe. Gram-positive cocci in clusters was seen on Gram-stain. Sputum was sent for culture and sensitivity. All other relevant investigations were normal.

Fine facial wrinkling, sparse sexual hair and breast atrophy, anemia and poor nutrition, hypotension and relative bradycardia (despite fever), hyponatremia and hypoglycemia pointed to the possibility of hypopituitarism.

A provisional diagnosis of community-acquired pneumonia (CAP) with severe euvolemic hyponatremia with high urine sodium and osmolality and possible hypopituitarism was made. She was started on intravenous antibiotics based on local protocol for CAP. She was given 3% saline for hyponatremia correction and dextrose infusion for hypoglycemia. Suspecting hypopituitarism, blood was sent for cortisol paired with adrenocorticotropic hormone (ACTH), thyroxine (T4), thyroid-stimulating hormone (TSH), luteinizing hormone (LH), follicle-stimulating hormone (FSH), prolactin, and insulin-like growth factor 1 (IGF-1). Then intravenous hydrocortisone 100 mg 6 hourly was initiated while laboratory reports were awaited. With antibiotics, saline, dextrose, and intravenous hydrocortisone she became conscious, oriented, and afebrile and could give a detailed history.

Her last child birth was 15 years back when she had delivered a full-term normal weight baby at home but was rushed to the hospital due to massive PPH. She remembers being very sick then and had received numerous units of blood transfusion at that time. She had lactational failure but did have some menstrual bleeding 3–4 times a few months after the birth of her last child after which she has been amenorrheic. She has always been weak ever since with asthenia, anorexia, and frequent postural symptoms. She was admitted on two more occasions earlier with hypotension and low sodium which improved with intravenous fluids.

Meanwhile, her endocrine reports came as follows: Serum cortisol 1.2 µg/dL, plasma ACTH 4.5 pg/mL, TSH 1.5 mIU/L, T4 3.6 µg/dL, serum LH 0.6 IU/mL, FSH 0.4 IU/mL, prolactin 2 ng/dL, and IGF-1 46 ng/mL suggesting a panhypopituitarism. MRI of the pituitary showed a completely empty sella.

A diagnosis of Sheehan's syndrome with panhypopituitarism was made. She was treated with intravenous hydrocortisone 100 mg 6 hourly which was gradually tapered. She was thereafter kept on a maintenance dose of oral hydrocortisone tablets 10 mg at 7 AM and 5 mg at 6 PM. She was started on 62.5 µg of levothyroxine (1.6 µg/kg) 3 days after start of hydrocortisone.

Case 2

A 30-year-old lady suffered massive PPH following the birth of her second baby by normal delivery. She complained of severe headache and vomiting and then lost consciousness. She was in hypovolemic shock and did not respond to resuscitative measures with blood transfusion, intravenous fluids, and inotropes, even if her vaginal bleeding was successfully controlled. She died 5 hours later. Autopsy revealed an enlarged grayish looking pituitary. Histopathological examination showed ischemic necrosis involving the entire anterior pituitary.

The postmortem findings suggested a pituitary apoplexy following massive PPH and a diagnosis of acute phase of Sheehan's syndrome was made.

DISCUSSION

Introduction

Sheehan's syndrome is postpartum pituitary failure due to pituitary infarction following massive PPH. Pituitary failure may be complete or partial; and acute or slowly progressive. The clinical presentation was described extensively by Harold L. Sheehan in 1937. However, pituitary necrosis on autopsy specimen of postpartum women was described as early as 1913 and 1914 by Glinsky and Simmons respectively.

Epidemiology and Demographics

The prevalence of Sheehan's syndrome varies in different regions of the world. Incidence is low in developed nations but higher in the developing nations due to domiciliary delivery and inadequate institutional obstetric care. In Kashmir, India, the prevalence of Sheehan's syndrome was estimated to be 3.1% of parous women ≥20 years of age and 63% of these women had delivery at home. One study from Turkey found Sheehan's syndrome to be the most common cause of hypopituitarism in women and Sheehan's syndrome was the 3rd most common cause of hypopituitarism in Philippines. Data from developed nations like USA, UK, and Japan showed the development of Sheehan's syndrome in postpartum women to be nil or very low. However, migration of women who delivered in their native countries to the developed world has increased the prevalence of Sheehan's in the developed nations. Therefore, physicians in both the developing and developed world need to be aware of this clinical entity which has a highly heterogeneous presentation.

In a study from Kolkata, India, the age of presentation ranged widely from 28 to 71 years. Another data from Turkey showed the typical age of presentation as 52.8 ± 12.3 years. The mean diagnostic delay can range from 7 to 27 years in studies from India, France, and Turkey. The delay is due to the nature of disease presentation which is typically nonspecific characterized by anorexia, asthenia, nausea, and postural symptoms; the overlooking or sometimes absence of typical symptoms like amenorrhea, lactational failure, and lack of awareness among physicians.

PATHOPHYSIOLOGY AND RISK FACTORS

The basic mechanism behind the development of postpartum pituitary infarction is the physiological enlargement of pituitary in pregnancy that predisposes it to ischemia due to increased vascular demand and/or compression of the vasculature by the enlarging pituitary gland. Following a PPH, hypovolemic shock-induced vasospasm of the arteries supplying the pituitary compromises the vascular supply of the enlarged pituitary which already has a precarious blood supply. Pregnant women who develop massive hemorrhage from other causes like gastrointestinal bleeding can develop pituitary infarction, suggesting that an enlarged pituitary with a compromised blood supply is required for its pathogenesis.

Nonpregnant individuals who develop massive hemorrhage do not develop pituitary infarction as the physiological demands of the pituitary are not increased. An exception is in the case of hematotoxic snake bite, where hemorrhagic necrosis of the normal-sized pituitary occurs along with massive bleeding at other sites. Toxins released from the hematotoxic snakes cause hemorrhage. This frequently results in hypopituitarism which can develop immediately or over the years. Hypopituitarism following hematotoxic snake bite is not an uncommon cause of hypopituitarism in endemic areas in India.

However, neither all patients with Sheehan's syndrome have a history of massive PPH nor do all patients with massive PPH develop Sheehan's syndrome. Thus, other factors contribute to pituitary infarction following PPH. These are small size sella, vasospasm, thrombosis, and clotting anomalies. In a study involving 114 patients with Sheehan's syndrome, the mean sella volume in patients with Sheehan's was 340.5 ± 214 mm^3 which was significantly lower than healthy women 602.5 ± 192 mm^3. When sella is small, the enlarged pituitary can easily compress the hypophyseal arteries against the sella turcica and the diaphragmatic sella compromising blood supply. Genetic mutations predisposing to procoagulant states are important risks for Sheehan's syndrome through thrombophilia and thrombosis. Important are mutations of coagulation factor V (F5), coagulation factor II (F2), methylenetetrahydrofolate reductase (MTHFR*C677T and MTHFR*A1298C), and plasminogen activator inhibitor type-1 (PAI-1).

Enlargement of the pituitary gland during pregnancy is contributed mainly by lactotroph hyperplasia which accounts for the increased prolactin levels in pregnancy, thereby preparing the breast for lactation. Studies have shown that in pregnancy there is decrease in the gonadotrophs and somatotrophs whereas the thyrotrophs and corticotrophs remain unchanged. In the first trimester, the pituitary enlarges by 45% and near term it is enlarged by 120–136%. The height of the pituitary increases from 4 to 8 mm to 10 mm at term and 12 mm in the immediate postpartum period. The pituitary comes back to prepregnancy size at around 6 months postpartum.

Certain characteristics of the vascular supply of the pituitary predisposes not only to infarction but specifically to involvement of certain areas of the pituitary. Briefly, the anatomy and blood supply of the pituitary can be described as follows. The pituitary which resides in the sella turcica has an anterior lobe (adenohypophysis) and a posterior lobe (neurohypophysis). The adenohypophysis has three parts: The pars distalis is the main component and secretes the anterior pituitary hormones, the pars intermediate is compressed in humans and the pars tuberalis surrounds the infundibulum or the stalk of the pituitary. The pars tuberalis, median eminence, and infundibulum receive blood supply from the superior hypophyseal artery and neurohypophysis receives blood supply from the inferior hypophyseal arteries; both of which arise (directly or indirectly) from the internal carotid artery. However, the blood supply of the pars distalis which is the main hormone producing area of the anterior pituitary is mostly via the venous drainage of the long and short portal veins. This unique circulation allows the pars distalis to receive hormones and substances from the hypothalamus, posterior pituitary, and periphery but predisposes it to ischemia. Lactotrophs and somatotrophs which are present in the lateral wings of the pituitary and dependent on portal (venous) circulation are mostly affected following a pituitary infarction. Corticotrophs and thyrotrophs are present in the median edge and the gonadotrophs are scattered throughout the pituitary. Their functions may, therefore, be completely or partially preserved for some time depending on the extent of the pituitary insult. Though rare, the posterior pituitary can also be involved resulting is diabetes insipidus (DI). But associated hypocortisolism and hypothyroidism can mask the polyuria and hypernatremia of DI which can be unmasked when hypocortisolism and hypothyroidism are treated.

Infarction leads to ischemic necrosis of the pituitary which is replaced subsequently by a fibrous scar with resultant volume loss. This produces a completely or a partially empty sella. Earlier authors had wrongly attributed the pituitary necrosis to puerperal sepsis. The destruction of the pituitary is not only chronic but also progressive. Thus, the presentation of the disease is both chronic and progressive (acute presentations, though rare are also seen as in Case 2). Over the years more pituitary cell lines can get affected. Therefore, it is difficult to explain the hormonal loss over the years to the acute insult at the time of disease initiation, and thus other factors are believed to be involved in the pathogenesis of this condition. Important among these is autoimmunity. The release of the normally sequestered pituitary antigens following ischemic necrosis can incite an autoimmune reaction that further accelerates the disease progression. A study from India showed that more women with Sheehan's syndrome (following PPH) had antibodies against pituitary antigens compared to normal women and postpartum women with hypopituitarism but no history of PPH. The antibody detected was against a 49-kDa pituitary cytosolic protein, neuron-specific enolase.

To summarize, Sheehan's syndrome occurs as a result of infarction of the enlarged pituitary due to massive PPH. Other factors predispose to pituitary ischemia and subsequent infarction. The pituitary destruction can be thought to have an acute initiation phase where a significant amount of the pituitary is destroyed by ischemic necrosis. This is followed over the ensuing years by a progressive phase of pituitary destruction where autoimmunity and possibly yet unknown factors contribute. If the initial phase cause massive necrosis, pituitary apoplexy can develop and this can be immediately fatal. More frequently the disease presents as a chronic progressive one with myriad clinical features.

Clinical Features

The classical criteria for the diagnosis of Sheehan's syndrome are: (1) Obstetrical history of severe PPH; (2) Severe hypotension or shock necessitating blood transfusion or fluid replacement; (3) Lactational failure; (4) Failure to resume regular menses after delivery; (5) Varying degree of anterior pituitary insufficiency; and (6) Partial or complete empty sella on imaging.

However, clinical features of Sheehan's syndrome are highly variable ranging from acute pituitary failure to the more common chronic progressive hypopituitarism with heterogeneous presentation. Sheehan himself noted the functional loss of the pituitary hormones was progressive but varied widely. He found that 17 of 112 women with complete glandular destruction at autopsy menstruated for varying periods, and 2 even had subsequent pregnancy. In a study of 114 women with Sheehan's syndrome, nonspecific symptoms were seen in >50% of affected women. The study also found higher incidence of complicated pregnancies in women who developed Sheehan's compared to baseline prevalence. The authors attributed their findings to the possibility of procoagulant states predisposing to both Sheehan's syndrome and pregnancy complications. In the same study 37.7% of the women reported breastfeeding normally for 15.1 ± 7 months; and while most (85.1%) had amenorrhea, 14.9% patients had regular menses for 32.2 ± 3.2 months after the last delivery. In a study from Kolkata, 94.4% patients had lactational failure; 72.2% did not menstruate after last child birth. Thus, lactational failure and amenorrhea though frequent are not sine qua non for the diagnosis of Sheehan's syndrome.

Acute presentation of Sheehan's (Case 2) in the immediate postpartum, though rare, can be fatal if not correctly diagnosed and treated. Patients present with features of pituitary apoplexy like headache, visual symptoms, loss of consciousness, and agalactia; and features of adrenal insufficiency like extreme fatigue, nausea, vomiting, hypotension, shock, hypoglycemia and hyponatremia. Posterior pituitary involvement can lead to DI.

Typically, Sheehan's has a chronic presentation and nonspecific symptoms dominate the clinical picture. The nonspecific symptoms are chronic ill-health, asthenia, anorexia, premature ageing, sleep disturbances, and mood disorders. If carefully searched for, most patients would have lactational failure, amenorrhea, and regression of secondary sexual characters. However, patients frequently are diagnosed in stressful condition that precipitates an acute adrenal insufficiency like surgery or severe infection as in our patient in Case 1.

Growth hormone and prolactin are the most commonly affected hormones whereas ACTH and TSH are among the last to be affected. This is explained by the distribution of the various pituitary cells and could be nature's way of preserving the hormones most vital for survival. It is, however, emphasized here again that there is no one way of involvement; and any combination and degree of hormone deficiency can occur in Sheehan's syndrome. The prevalence of ACTH and TSH deficiency ranges from 80% to 100% in various studies. Though rare, the posterior pituitary can be involved. DI can occur in 5% and partial DI can occur in one-third of patients. Coexisting hypocortisolism and hypothyroidism can mask the features of DI. Bone loss occurs in Sheehan's syndrome and multiple pituitary hormone deficiency is a strong contributory factor.

When patients with (chronic) Sheehan's syndrome present acutely, they often do so because of adrenal crisis (Case 1). Frequently, there is a stressful condition which precipitates adrenal crisis in a patient with latent ACTH deficiency. Deficiency of other anterior pituitary hormones like thyrotropin and growth hormone frequently deteriorates the clinical picture. Hyponatremia is the most frequent electrolyte disturbance in patients with Sheehan's syndrome ranging from 21% to 59%. Adrenal insufficiency and hypothyroidism cause hyponatremia by decreasing free water clearance. Increased antidiuretic hormone (ADH) worsens hyponatremia and it can occur because of the stimulation of its release by corticotropin-releasing hormone (CRH), hypovolemia-induced ADH release and acute illness (e.g., pneumonia) related syndrome of inappropriate antidiuretic hormone secretion (SIADH). The hyponatremia is a euvolemic hyponatremia with high urine osmolality and sodium like SIADH. Thus, in all cases of suspected SIADH, thyroid and adrenal function must be assessed. Hypoglycemia is another important finding. One study found Sheehan's syndrome to be the second most common cause of hypoglycemia. Adrenal insufficiency, hypothyroidism, growth hormone deficiency, and poor nutritional intake all contribute to the hypoglycemia. The presence of hyponatremia and hypoglycemia in a hypotensive patient (sometimes in shock), with anemia, facial wrinkling and loss of secondary sexual characters suggest hypopituitarism. If a history of PPH is available, Sheehan's syndrome is established; and this can be confirmed by relevant laboratory and imaging reports.

Diagnosis

Laboratory Investigation

In patients presenting acutely blood sample for ACTH and cortisol should be drawn before urgent resuscitation. They will be found to be low. T4, TSH, LH, FSH, IGF-1, and prolactin can all be low. Patients often have hyponatremia and hypoglycemia.

Prolactin and growth hormone are the most commonly affected hormones but as mentioned before there is no specific pattern of hormonal loss. The progressive nature of the disease means that more hormones may be affected over the ensuing years. Low basal levels of prolactin suggest prolactin deficiency. In patients with amenorrhea, low or normal basal LH and FSH levels suggest central hypogonadism. This will be accompanied by low basal estradiol (E2) levels.

Low morning (8–9 AM) serum cortisol with low or normal ACTH levels suggests central hypocortisolism. Morning serum cortisol below 3 µg/dL confirms cortisol deficiency and this along with a low or normal ACTH confirms secondary adrenal insufficiency. Morning basal cortisol >18 µg/dL confirms cortisol sufficiency but in those with cortisol between 3 and 18 µg/dL stimulation tests are needed to test the ACTH reserve. Stimulation tests commonly performed are ACTH stimulation tests and insulin tolerance test (ITT). It should be kept in mind that the ACTH stimulation test may be normal if Sheehan's is of recent onset (<6 weeks) as the adrenals have not yet atrophied and would therefore respond to exogenous ACTH. During ITT, in normal persons, serum cortisol increases to ≥18 µg/dL when the serum glucose falls to <50 mg/dL. Insulin tolerance test is the gold standard but is contraindicated in patients with seizures and ischemic heart disease. Other tests to detect ACTH reserve are glucagon stimulation test, measurement of overnight metyrapone stimulation, and CRH testing.

Low thyroxine and low or normal TSH concentrations confirms the diagnosis of central hypothyroidism in the absence of nonthyroidal illness. The symptoms of central hypothyroidism are similar to but less severe than primary hypothyroidism and there is absence of a goiter. Sometimes, the TSH levels may be slightly increased in central hypothyroidism due to sialylation of TSH that prolongs its half-life but decreases its biological activity.

Low IGF-1 levels with at least three anterior pituitary hormone deficiencies are conclusive diagnosis of growth hormone deficiency and no further testing is required. Stimulation testing is done to document growth hormone deficiency in other situations. ITT is the gold standard. Other tests are growth hormone-releasing hormone (GHRH), arginine, clonidine, levodopa (L-DOPA), and the combination of arginine and L-DOPA stimulation testing.

Posterior pituitary involvement with (ADH) deficiency can occur in Sheehan's syndrome. The clinical picture may be masked by coexisting hypocortisolism and hypothyroidism. DI causes polyuria (>3 L/day) and can be confirmed by water deprivation test. A urine osmolality of <300 mOsmol/kg in the presence of fluid deprivation and subsequent response to arginine vasopressin (AVP) is suggestive of central DI. Copeptin, the C-terminal moiety of AVP is a stable marker of AVP concentrations. A combination of a fluid deprivation test with hypertonic saline challenge using copeptin measurements provides an accurate diagnosis in 96% of patients presenting with polyuria and polydipsia.

The most common electrolyte abnormality is hyponatremia. Other electrolyte abnormalities like hypokalemia, hypomagnesemia, hypocalcemia, and hypophosphatemia have been reported. Patients typically have normocytic normochromic anemia, thrombocytopenia, and sometimes pancytopenia. Coagulation abnormalities are also reported.

Imaging

Pituitary MRI shows a completely or a partially empty sella in around 70% and 30% of individual with Sheehan's syndrome respectively. Progressive atrophy of the gland following the initial ischemic necrosis produces this picture. Rarely, normal looking pituitary gland has been reported. In acute Sheehan's syndrome, a non-hemorrhagic enlarged pituitary with a small rim of gadolinium enhancement is seen. The pituitary is enlarged much more than would be expected in a normal gestation.

Management

If after the control of postpartum hemorrhage, and after adequate intravenous fluids replacement and blood transfusion a woman remains hypotensive, acute phase of Sheehan's should be suspected (Case 2). She should be evaluated and treated for adrenal insufficiency immediately; evaluation of other hormonal deficiencies can be deferred until 4 to 6 weeks postpartum. Immediate management of secondary adrenal insufficiency includes injection hydrocortisone 100 mg 6 hourly and dextrose and saline infusion. Dose will be adjusted based on clinical and biochemical monitoring of the patient.

Replacement of deficient hormones and regular screening for new deficiencies form the basis of treatment in the chronic phase of Sheehan's syndrome. Importantly, management of other complications of hypopituitarism like cardiometabolic and bone health is important to improve morbidity and mortality outcomes. Mortality is higher in Sheehan's syndrome by 1.2–2.7 times.

The replacement of cortisol deficiency is the most important aspect of the hormone replacement. Hydrocortisone or cortisone acetate (where available) are preferred. Aim of replacement is to provide a daily dose that would be physiological and mimic the circadian serum cortisol profile. Studies have shown that the mean cortisol production in healthy individuals is 15.5–19 mg/day and adverse metabolic effects have been seen in hypopituitarism receiving >20 mg/day. So, the daily dose should never be >30 mg/day and should be much lower than that. Patients with partial deficiency can be advised low dose (5–10 mg/day) or stress dose of hydrocortisone. Patients should be advised to double their dose of glucocorticoids during an illness and a steroid card must be provided. All patients should have an emergency kit of parenteral hydrocortisone administration. Monitoring should look for clinical features of glucocorticoid excess or deficiency supported by laboratory reports of electrolytes and glucose. Addition of 20–50 mg of dehydroepiandrosterone (DHEA) may improve well-being and libido.

Levothyroxine replacement should be given only after the patient has had adequate glucocorticoid replacement for at least few days, otherwise an adrenal crisis can be precipitated. This is because thyroid hormone replacement increases demand and clearance of cortisol. The typical dose is 1.6 µg/day and the starting dose and dose titration should be chosen with caution in all elderly patients and in those ischemic heart disease. Monitoring is to be done by assessing T4 or free thyroxine (FT4) concentration with blood drawn before the morning dose of levothyroxine.

In women <50 years (usual age of menopause), estrogen and cyclic progesterone are often given in the absence of contraindications (deep vein thrombosis, pulmonary embolism, cirrhosis of liver, acute hepatitis and uncontrolled hypertension). Younger women need higher dose of estrogen whereas lower doses are needed in older women. Transdermal estrogen compared to oral estrogen causes less effect on lipids, coagulation, inflammation, and levels of binding proteins. Gonadotropins have been tried for fertility with successful pregnancy in few cases. Regular follow-up and adjustment of glucocorticoid dose is necessary once patient becomes pregnant.

Opinion is mixed on the use of growth hormone in Sheehan's syndrome. Studies have shown that growth hormone replacement improves body composition and cardiometabolic health. The dose in adult is low and dose adjustment is done by titrating the IGF-1 levels to the normal age adjusted levels every 4–6 weeks. Oral estrogen replacement attenuates serum IGF-1 response to growth hormone. If oral estrogen is withdrawn or replaced by transdermal estrogen growth hormone, dose reduction is required. Growth hormone treatment can unmask central hypothyroidism and central adrenal insufficiency and therefore thyroid and adrenal function needs to be monitored in individuals started on growth hormone; and dose adjustments may be needed in individuals already on levothyroxine and glucocorticoid replacement.

For the treatment of DI, desmopressin tablets in two or three divided daily doses, or nasal preparations one to two times daily are used. When administered nasally, antidiuretic effects of desmopressin start between 6 and 12 hours. When switching to oral from intranasal, oral desmopressin should start at least 12 hours after the last intranasal dose.

Differential Diagnosis

Two important differential diagnosis of Sheehan's syndrome are lymphocytic hypophysitis and bleeding in a pre-existing pituitary adenoma.

Acutely lymphocytic hypophysitis can present with headache, visual symptoms, and hypopituitarism; in the chronic stage lymphocytic hypo-physitis can lead to empty sella with hypopituitarism. It may be difficult to differentiate these features from the acute and chronic presentations of Sheehan's syndrome. Distinguishing features from Sheehan's syndrome are absence of severe PPH, history of autoimmunity, presence of DI, hyper-prolactinemia, and some imaging characteristics in lymphocytic hypo-physitis. MRI findings in lymphocytic hypophysitis are pituitary and infundibular enlargement with symmetrical and homogenous gadolinium enhancement, loss of the posterior pituitary bright spot, and presence of a dura tail.

Bleeding into a pre-existing adenoma in the postpartum period may mimic acute Sheehan's syndrome. Proper history and imaging features can differentiate the two. History of massive PPH suggest Sheehan's syndrome. An enlarged pituitary on imaging can be seen in both conditions; but an enlarged pituitary with a wide sella would suggest a pre-existing adenoma. Spontaneous shrinkage of the pituitary mass after a few months and absence of local invasion suggest Sheehan's syndrome.

Coming Back to Our Patients

Case 1: The patient improved following hydrocortisone and levothyroxine replacement. She was also given oral estrogen and progesterone preparation, after contraindications to their use were ruled out. Growth hormone was not given due to cost issue and reluctance to daily injections. She was also provided calcium and vitamin D supplementation. Her cardiometabolic health was assessed and she was found to be dyslipidemic with high low-density lipoprotein cholesterol (LDL-C), triglycerides, and low high-density lipoprotein cholesterol (HDL-C) and was started on atorvastatin 20 mg/day at bedtime.

Case 2: This case highlights the importance of heightened awareness about the acute phase of Sheehan's syndrome among the treating physicians. Acute resuscitative measures with hydrocortisone, intravenous saline, and dextrose could be life-saving.

Prevention

The awareness of this condition is the first step in its prevention. Discouraging home deliveries and providing adequate obstetric care are vital. The possibility of an acute Sheehan's in a women who do not respond to resuscitative measures following a PPH should be kept in mind and should be managed accordingly. All women who survived a PPH should be followed up regularly for pituitary function assessment, so that she may never present in a crisis. Guidelines for follow-up of such women must be well established as for women with a history of gestational diabetes mellitus.

CONCLUSION

Sheehan's syndrome is not a rare cause of hypopituitarism in developing countries. The disease is chronic and progressive, and more pituitary hormones can be affected over the years. Diagnosis is often missed because of nonspecific symptoms and lack of physician awareness; and patients frequently present in an acute state. Adequate obstetric care, recognition of acute phase and follow-up of all women with PPH can improve outcomes. Sufficient hormone replacements are available which can improve the quality of life of affected women.

SUGGESTED READINGS

1. Diri H, Karaca Z, Tanriverdi F, et al. Sheehan's syndrome: new insights into an old disease. Endocrine. 2016;51(1):22-31.
2. Keleştimur F. Sheehan's syndrome. Pituitary. 2003;6(4):181-8.
3. Kilicli F, Dokmetas HS, Acibucu F. Sheehan's syndrome. Gynecol Endocrinol. 2013;29(4): 292-5.
4. Krysiak R, Okopień B. Zespół Sheehana—zapomniana choroba ze stuletnia historia [Sheehan's syndrome—a forgotten disease with 100 years' history]. Przegl Lek. 2015;72(6):313-20.
5. Laway BA, Baba MS. Sheehan syndrome. J Pak Med Assoc. 2021;71(4):1282-12568.
6. Matsuwaki T, Khan KN, Inoue T, et al. Evaluation of obstetrical factors related to Sheehan syndrome. J Obstet Gynaecol Res. 2014;40(1):46-52.
7. Tessnow AH, Wilson JD. The changing face of Sheehan's syndrome. Am J Med Sci. 2010;340(5): 402-6.

4

CHAPTER

Raynaud's Phenomenon in Acromegaly: An Unusual Presentation

Shikha Gupta, Harika Mandava, Bindu Kulshreshtha

INTRODUCTION

Acromegaly is a disorder characterized by increased Growth Hormone secretion after the fusion of epiphysis is complete. Apart from clinical features associated with an enlarging pituitary mass, the presenting features of the disorder are usually subtle involving soft tissue overgrowth or coarsened clinical features. While acromegaly patients are prone to cardiovascular morbidity, Raynaud's phenomenon involving small vessels of the hands is exceedingly rare. Here we describe a young male who had Raynaud's phenomenon and was later diagnosed to have acromegaly.

CASE HISTORY

A 33-year-old male was accompanying his sister, a Turner's syndrome patient, when the doctor noticed his acromegaloid features. On interrogation, he revealed that there had been change in his facial features over the past 4 years. He also noticed broadening of his hands and fingers and his previous rings did not fit now. He also noticed discoloration of distal fingers and hands to white and then to blue on exposure to cold/especially in winters. There was no history of headache or galactorrhea or any history of autoimmune disorders. He had backache that did not interfere with his daily routine or require oral medications. There was no history of rash, oral ulcers or photo sensitivity.

Examination revealed a normotensive patient, height of 174 cm with frontal bossing, fleshy nose, bulbous lips, and broadened hands and feet (**Fig. 1**). Pallor and cyanosis of distal fingers and hands on exposure to cold was noted (**Fig. 2**) that normalized when exposed to normal room temperature. Neurologic examination was normal. Hemogram, blood glucose, lipid profile, liver and kidney function tests were normal. Post glucose growth hormone (GH) levels were high (19.1 ng/dL). MRI pituitary revealed a 4 mm pituitary microadenoma. Prolactin, thyroid profile, and cortisol levels were normal however testosterone levels were low (3.98 nmol/L) with normal luteinizing

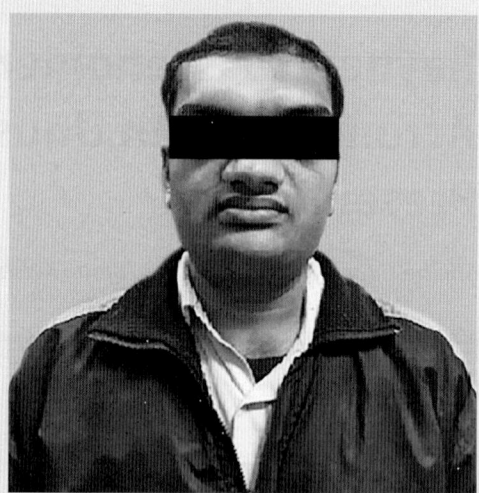

FIG. 1: Patient with facial acromegaloid features. (***For color version, see plate 1***)

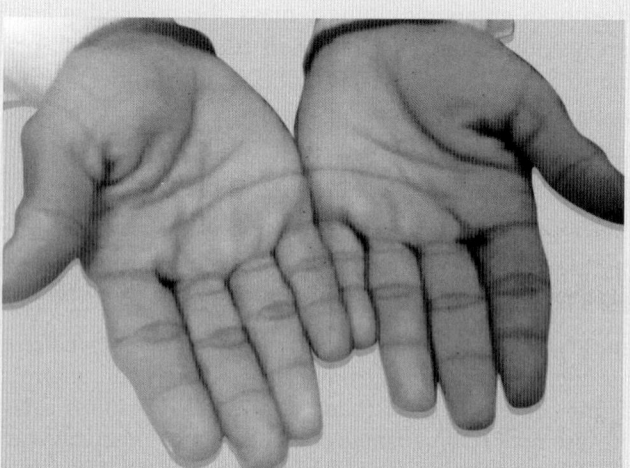

FIG. 2: Both hands showing Raynaud's phenomenon (demarcation line between discolored and normal portion). (***For color version, see plate 1***)

hormone (LH) and follicle-stimulating hormone (FSH) levels. Investigation for back pain revealed normal calcium but low 25(OH) vitamin D levels (11.5 ng/mL). X-ray lumbosacral spine revealed degenerative changes. Coagulation profile [Prothrombin Time (PT) and Partial Thromboplastin Time with Kaolin (PTTK)] was normal. RA factor and ANA levels were negative. Echocardiography revealed a grade I diastolic dysfunction with ejection fraction of 60%. Color Doppler of the upper limb vessels revealed a generalized decrease in peak systolic velocity in the ulnar and radial artery, multiple peaks during diastole and diminished diastolic high resistance flow. Patient was advised surgery but he refused and was started on injection octreotide long-acting release (LAR) 20 µg subcutaneous (sc) once a month. Patient is doing well with injection. For Raynaud's phenomenon he was asked to avoid cold and other stress factors.

DISCUSSION

Acromegaly

Acromegaly is a hormonal disorder characterized by excess growth hormone (GH) after the growth plates have closed. Overproduction of GH can be due to pituitary tumor or ectopic production of GH from nonpituitary tumors. In about 95% of cases, the excess production of GH is due to benign tumor, i.e., pituitary adenoma. Most GH secreting pituitary tumors arise spontaneously and are not genetically inherited. These tumors can cause compression of surrounding tissue as they grow larger and alter production of other hormones like prolactin, cortisol, and thyroid. Elevated serum prolactin levels with or without galactorrhea can be seen in 30% of patients. Rarely, acromegaly may be caused by excess secretion of GH from tumors of pancreas, lung, and adrenal glands. These extrapituitary tumors either release GH themselves or more frequently they produce growth hormone–releasing hormone (GHRH) that stimulates pituitary to make GH. Middle-aged adults are most commonly affected by acromegaly.

Symptomatology

Pituitary adenoma producing GH can have varied presentations depending on the rate of GH production and tumor progression. Younger patients tend to have more aggressive tumors. The term "Acro+megaly" in Greek is "extremities and enlargement" which reflects one of its most common symptoms. Patient often notices changes in ring and shoe size due to abnormal growth of hands and feet. Enlargement of hands and feet is often an early feature. Overgrowth of bone and cartilage occurs which leads to alteration of facial features like protrusion of brow and lower jaw, enlargement of nasal bone, and spacing of teeth. When tissue thickens, it may trap nerves causing carpal tunnel syndrome, which results in numbness and weakness in hands. Other symptoms includes joint pains, thick coarse oily skin, skin tags, enlarged nose, lips and tongue, deepening of voice, headaches and impaired vision due to compression by tumor, erectile dysfunction in men, menstrual irregularities, and galactorrhea in women.

Complications of acromegaly include arthritis and carpal tunnel syndrome, enlarged heart, liver fibrosis and bile duct hyperplasia, hypertension, diabetes mellitus, heart failure, kidney failure, and colorectal cancer. Compression of the optic chiasm can cause bitemporal hemianopia.

Diagnosis

Diagnosis of acromegaly is done by GH suppression test and insulin-like growth factor 1 (IGF-1) levels. GH suppression test is done with 75–100 g of glucose which suppresses GH level to <1 ng/mL within 1 hour of glucose loading in normal individual. In people with GH overproduction, this suppression does not occur. IGF-1 level also rises as GH increases hepatic production of IGF-1. Elevated IGF-1 levels almost always indicate acromegaly except in pregnant women. After blood tests, contrast-enhanced MRI scan of pituitary is done to locate and detect size of the tumor. If MRI head remains normal then GHRH estimation and CT scan of possible tumor sites should be done. Other anterior pituitary axis should also be evaluated as part of work up. This includes serum prolactin, thyroid stimulating hormone (TSH), gonadotropic hormones (FSH, LH), and adrenocorticotropic hormone (ACTH). Other biochemical investigations include hemogram (to look for polycythemia), blood glucose in the fasting and postprandial state, liver and kidney function tests. Other investigations include colonoscopy to look for colonic polyps, 2D echocardiography (to look for hypertrophic cardiomyopathy) and perimetry.

Management

Treatment modalities of acromegaly are surgical removal of the tumors, medical therapy, and radiation therapy. Transsphenoidal surgery is the first option recommended for most people with acromegaly as it is often a rapid and effective treatment. Tumors which are smaller in size (<5 mm) and confined within sella with preoperative serum GH level <40 µg/L portend favorable surgical outcome. Postoperatively 90% of patients with microadenoma achieve GH level lower than 2.5 µg/L and <50% of all sized macroadenoma achieve GH level lower than 2 µg/L. Current medical treatment of acromegaly include somatostatin analog octreotide or lanreotide. These are somatotropin release inhibiting factor (SRIF) analogs which predominantly binds to somatostatin receptor 2 (SSTR2) receptors and inhibits GH secretion with potency greater than native SRIF and are effective in lowering GH and IGF-1 level in 50–70% of patients. These long-acting drugs must be injected every 4 weeks. Another drug used is GH receptor antagonist, i.e., pegvisomant. These drugs get bound to GH receptor and block peripheral GH action. However, they do not target the pituitary tumor. Dopamine agonists like bromocriptine and cabergoline are used either as primary or adjuvant therapy in acromegalic patients especially with mildly elevated GH and IGF-1 levels. Radiation therapy has been used both as primary treatment or in combination with surgery and drugs. It is usually reserved for patients who have residual tumor even after surgery and are not responding to medical treatment. Up to 5,000 RADS are administered in split doses of 180 radiation fractions divided over 6 weeks. Radiation therapy arrests tumor growth and most pituitary adenomas ultimately shrink, however, a long period of time usually years are needed to achieve reduction in tumor growth.

Raynaud's Phenomenon

Raynaud's phenomenon is a clinical condition characterized by episodes of vasospasm in hands and foot parts due to cold or emotional stress which may result in a reversible pain and color change manifesting in the form of a pallor, erythematosis or cyanosis of digits. Symptoms of Raynaud's phenomenon includes paresthesia, abnormal sensation of coldness or burning pain, periodic color changes in one or more digits in response to a cold condition, emotional stress, and vibration. These changes are usually reversible. In severe cases, these changes may result in a localized ischemia and ulceration.

It is of two types: Primary Raynaud's, when the cause is unknown and secondary Raynaud's which occur as a result of another condition like occupational effect, hematological influence, autoimmune disorder (systemic sclerosis), acromegaly, Fabry's disease, pheochromocytoma, pulmonary adenocarcinoma, and myxedema.

Vasospasm duration in primary Raynaud's may range from few minutes to hours and usually without any significant effect such as tissue loss while in secondary Raynaud's vasospasm may be associated with inflamed digital gangrene and infected finger ulcers.

There is an increased effect of $\alpha2$-adrenergic response that stimulates vasospasm in Raynaud's phenomenon although mechanism is not fully understood. More than 80% of Raynaud's phenomenon is of primary type and in 20% of the affected patients, there may an underlying cause of the disease like systemic sclerosis, acromegaly, Fabry's disease.

The prevalence of Raynaud phenomenon ranges from 3 to 5%, with women more commonly affected than men. Younger people are more commonly affected as compared to older ones.

Pathophysiology

Raynaud's phenomenon is probably due to an imbalance between vaso-constriction and vasodilation mechanism, which results from impairment in neural regulations of vascular tone, with the circulation of chemical mediators. Altered or impaired vasodilation may also cause Raynaud phenomenon. Chemical mediators involved in vasoconstriction are maintained by vasodilators which includes nitric oxide and prostaglandins. The outcome of secondary Raynaud phenomenon in affected patients is influenced by prostaglandins which causes an increase in the fibrinolysis. The pathogenesis of Raynaud syndrome is stimulated by decrease in vasodilatory chemical mediators such as nitric oxide. Among patients having secondary Raynaud's phenomenon, endothelin-1 a potent vaso-constrictor has been found to be in high amount. Increased episode of fibrosis and structural changes in blood vessels have also been observed in the patients with increased circulatory levels of the endothelin-1 mediators. A neuropeptide called calcitonin is an active vasodilator released by the nerves that regulate blood supply in the vessels.

Most often, Raynaud phenomenon is commonly diagnosed clinically. Clinically, both primary and secondary types are differentiated based on the symptoms and by special technique (vascular imaging studies) including laboratory investigations such as blood screening.

Treatment of Raynaud phenomenon depends on the type or form of the syndrome. Primary Raynaud phenomenon may not often require pharmacological therapy since it may be reversed by the removal of inciting agent, however most secondary forms are better managed with drugs such as dihydroxypyridine (nifedipine) and prazosin.

Discussion Related to Coassociation of Acromegaly and Raynaud's Phenomenon in Our Patient

Raynaud's phenomenon has rarely been described in patients with acromegaly. Some in vitro experiments on the subcutaneous tissue have revealed that GH has direct effects on vasculature. GH may stimulate in vitro proliferation of vascular smooth muscle cell which leads to hypertrophic remodeling of vessel wall, also there is embarrassed endothelial function due to reduced nitric oxide and endothelium-derived hyperpolarizing factor bioavailability. This could be the background for developing vascular phenomenon like hypertension or Raynaud's phenomenon in acromegaly patients.

Maison et al. compared cutaneous vasoactivity responses by laser Doppler flowmetry at hand in 10 acromegaly patients and 10 normal controls. The warm test and ischemia release induced an increase in both dorsal and palmar skin perfusion, but reactivities in acromegalic patients were about one-half of those measured in controls; Cold pressor test resulted in significant decreases in both cutaneous flows ($p < 0.01$) in the two groups, with a larger vasoconstriction in acromegalic patients as compared with controls. They concluded that endothelium-dependent vasodilation appears to be impaired while sympathetic-mediated vasoconstrictive response is increased in patients with acromegaly. We also observed a flow pattern consistent with a high resistance flow in our subject similar to the above mentioned study. In conclusion, this was a rare presentation of Raynaud's phenomenon in our subject with acromegaly.

CONCLUSION

This patient was not aware about his condition and was undiagnosed till he visited us where he was diagnosed with acromegaly on the basis of observation of enlargement of extremities. On further interrogation, he told that he had bluish discoloration of extremities on exposure to cold which was suggestive of Raynaud's phenomenon. So while managing acromegalic patients, we should also inquire about symptoms of Raynaud's phenomenon.

SUGGESTED READINGS

1. Bunker CB , Goldsmith PC, Leslie TA, Hayes N, Foreman JC, Dowd PM. Calcitonin gene-related peptide, endothelin-1, the cutaneous microvasculature and Raynaud's phenomenon. Br J Dermatol. 1996; 134(3):399-406.

2. Khaleh B, Matucci-Cerinic M. Raynaud's phenomenon and scleroderma. Dysregulated neuroendothelial control of vascular tone. Arthritis Rheum. 1995;38(1):1-4.

3. Lugo G, Pena L, Cordido F. Clinical Manifestations and Diagnosis of Acromegaly. Int J Endocrinol. 2012;2012:540398.

4. Maison P, Démolis P, Young J, et al. Vascular reactivity in acromegalic patients: preliminary evidence for regional endothelial dysfunction and increased sympathetic vasoconstriction. Clin Endocrinol (Oxf). 2000;53(4):445-51.

5. Melmed S, Polonsky KS, Larsen PR, Kronenberg HM. Pituitary masses and Tumours. Williams Textbook of Endocrinology, 13th edition. Amsterdam: Elsevier; 2016. p. 268-85.

6. Melmed S. Acromegaly. N Engl J Med. 2006;355:2558-73.

7. Muhammad A, van der Lely AJ, Neggers SJ. Review of current and emerging treatment in acromegaly. Neth J Med. 2015;73(8):362-70.

8. Paisley AN, Izzard AS, Gemmell I, et al. Small vessel remodeling and impaired endothelial-dependent dilatation in subcutaneous resistance arteries from patients with acromegaly. J Clin Endocrinol Metab. 2009;94(4):1111-7.

9. Rajagopalan S, Pfenninger D, Chakrabarti A, et al. Increased asymmetric dimethylarginine and endothelin 1 levels in secondary Raynaud's phenomenon: implications for vascular dysfunction and progression of disease. Arthritis Rheum. 2003;48(7):1992-2000.

10. Rizzoni D, Porteri E, Giustina A, et al. Acromegalic patients show the presence of hypertrophic remodeling of subcutaneous small resistance arteries. Hypertension. 2004;43(3):561-5.

5 Approach to a Case of Hyperprolactinemia

CHAPTER

Saba Samad Memon, Mukesh Kumar Srivastava, Mohd Ashraf Ganie

INTRODUCTION

Elevated levels of serum prolactin, an anterior pituitary hormone, can have varied clinical presentation from asymptomatic to hypogonadotropic hypogonadism and infertility. Markedly elevated levels usually signify a prolactin-secreting adenoma. Management of hyperprolactinemia depends on correcting the underlying etiology. Dopamine agonists like bromocriptine and cabergoline are the first line agents in treatment of prolactinomas.

CASE HISTORY

A 28-year-old male patient, resident of Bihar, presented with complaints of headache for the last 2 years. The headache was severe, bilateral, not relieved by analgesics and not associated with vomiting, photophobia or phonophobia. The headache was present on almost every day and was usually worse in the morning. He also complained of visual field loss since the last 2 months, which was gradual, painless, and progressive loss of both temporal fields (right more than left). He had no history of seizures, altered sensorium, or focal neurological deficit. He had undergone MRI of brain for his complaints which revealed pituitary tumor for which he was referred to endocrinology. He had no history of impotence, decreased libido, infertility, weight gain, or increase in size of hands or feet. He had no significant past history. Family history was unremarkable. He denied history of addiction or intake of any drugs.

His general physical examination was within normal limits. He had decreased temporal visual fields bilaterally. There was no papilledema. There was no galactorrhea, thyroid gland was not palpable and secondary sexual characteristics were well preserved. Rest of systemic examination was unremarkable.

His investigations revealed elevated serum prolactin 3798 ng/mL, thyroid stimulating hormone (TSH) 2.4 U/mL, growth hormone (GH) 0.314 µg/L, adrenocorticotropic hormone (ACTH) 36.8 pg/mL, and cortisol 12 µg/dL.

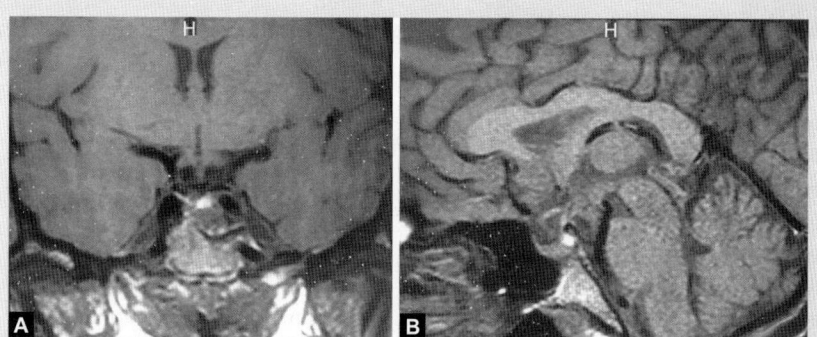

FIGS. 1A AND B: Contrast-enhanced MRI of brain in coronal and sagittal view showing 1.1 cm pituitary tumor.

His liver and renal functions were within normal limits. MRI of brain (**Figs. 1A and B**) was reviewed and reported as 1.1 cm mass lesion on left side of pituitary with sellar extension. A formal visual field examination was done to confirm bitemporal hemianopia.

In view of symptomatic prolactinoma, he was started on cabergoline 0.25 mg once a week. He was cautioned about possibility of side effects like nausea and hypotension. On follow-up, prolactin levels had declined to 2,950 ng/mL. Hence, cabergoline was increased to 0.25 mg twice a week. Serial measurement of prolactin levels and MRI to look for resolution in size of macroadenoma were planned for him.

DISCUSSION

Hyperprolactinemia is a common clinical problem, more so in women with reproductive issues. Prolactin is a polypeptide hormone secreted by lactotropes from anterior pituitary. It is predominantly under tonic inhibition by hypothalamic dopamine. Dopamine produced by arcuate nuclei of hypothalamus reach the lactotrope through hypothalamic hypophyseal portal vessels which traverse through the pituitary stalk. Other factors which regulate prolactin secretion include inhibitory mediators like gamma-aminobutyric acid (GABA), acetylcholine, somatostatin, norepinephrine, and stimulatory mediators like thyrotropin-releasing hormone (TRH), estrogen, vasoactive intestinal peptide (VIP), oxytocin, serotonin, etc. The main effects of prolactin include its role in milk production during pregnancy and lactation. Excessive levels of prolactin suppress gonadotropin secretion.

Etiology

The etiology of hyperprolactinemia (**Box 1**) can be broadly divided as physiological, diseases of hypothalamus and pituitary, drug induced, and systemic disorders.

BOX 1 | **Causes of hyperprolactinemia.**

Physiological
- Pregnancy
- Lactation
- Sleep
- Stress
- Coitus
- Exercise

Diseases of hypothalamus and pituitary
- Hypothalamic tumors: Craniopharyngioma, meningioma, dysgerminoma, metastatic breast carcinoma
- Infiltrative diseases of hypothalamus: Sarcoidosis, histiocytosis, other granulomatous disorders
- Irradiation to hypothalamus
- Rathke's cleft cyst
- Disruption of pituitary stalk: Head trauma, sellar surgery, suprasellar extension of pituitary mass
- Pituitary tumors: Prolactinoma, macroadenoma, plurihormonal adenoma, thyrotropinomas, metastasis
- Acromegaly
- Hypothyroidism
- Infiltrative diseases of pituitary, lymphocytic hypophysitis

Systemic disorders
- Chronic renal failure
- Cirrhosis
- Polycystic ovary syndrome
- Seizures
- Pseudocyesis
- Neurogenic: Chest wall trauma, herpes zoster, chest surgery
- Ectopic production: Renal cell carcinoma, ovarian teratoma, gonadoblastoma, non-Hodgkin lymphoma, etc.

Drug induced
- Dopamine antagonists: Chlorpromazine, haloperidol, risperidone, metoclopramide, domperidone
- Dopamine depletors and synthesis inhibitors: Reserpine, verapamil
- Others: Estrogens, ranitidine, opioids, phenytoin, amitriptyline

---

Physiological causes: Prolactin levels rise throughout pregnancy, with peak levels at delivery. There is increase in size of pituitary gland and prolactin-producing lactotropes during pregnancy. The levels of prolactin in pregnancy can be as high as 200–500 ng/mL (mean of 207 ng/mL). These decline after delivery to almost normal levels at 6 weeks postpartum despite continued breastfeeding. Suckling causes an episodic rise in prolactin levels. However, nipple stimulation or breast examination in nonlactating women and men does not increase prolactin levels markedly. The increase in prolactin levels, seen during sleep, returns to normal in an hour after awakening. Stress (e.g., psychological stress, physical discomfort, exercise, myocardial infarction, etc.) can also increase prolactin levels, more so in women. The levels of prolactin due to stress are usually <40 ng/mL.

Any disease that interferes with secretion and transport of dopamine from hypothalamus to pituitary can result in hyperprolactinemia, e.g., tumors or infiltrative diseases of hypothalamus, pituitary stalk section, cranial irradiation, etc. These, however, rarely cause elevation of prolactin to levels beyond 100 ng/mL. Lactotrope adenomas (prolactinomas) are the most important cause of prolactin levels beyond 200 ng/mL. They comprise 30–40% of all pituitary adenomas. They are usually sporadic, although can be seen in MEN 1 syndrome. They are usually benign. Prolactinoma can be microadenoma (<1 cm) or macroadenoma (>1 cm). Serum prolactin levels correlate to the size of the tumor. Those <1 cm usually have levels below 200 ng/mL; between 1 and 2 cm have 200–1,000 ng/mL; while adenomas greater than 2 cm in diameter have prolactin levels above 1,000 ng/mL. Discrepancy between adenoma size and prolactin values may be found in not well-differentiated adenomas, artifact in prolactin measurement or adenomas with a largely cystic component. Plurihormonal adenomas may secrete prolactin as well as another hormone like GH, ACTH, and rarely TSH. Nonfunctioning pituitary tumors can also cause hyperprolactinemia by stalk compression. Hypothyroidism can cause elevation in prolactin levels in 20% cases, even if it is subclinical. Hypothyroidism may mediate this increase through elevated TRH levels. Acromegaly has been associated with hyperprolactinemia in 50% cases.

Chronic renal failure and dialysis have been associated with an increase in prolactin levels due to decreased renal clearance. It returns to normal after transplantation. Elevation of prolactin in polycystic ovary syndrome (PCOS) may be due to increased estrogen levels. The pathogenesis of hyperprolactinemia in cirrhosis is unknown. Stimulation of neural pathways like chest wall trauma, herpes, etc., can lead to elevation in prolactin levels. Ectopic production of prolactin by tumors is very rare.

Drugs should be kept as an important differential of hyperprolactinemia. Dopamine antagonists mainly used as antipsychotics are frequently implicated. Haloperidol, phenothiazines, and risperidone are major culprits. Risperidone can cause prolactin levels as high as 200 ng/mL. Prokinetics like metoclopramide and domperidone, and antihistamines like ranitidine are most frequently prescribed drugs and should always be ruled out. The presence of drug as an implicating factor does not necessarily rule out other causes. Return of levels to normal after stopping of offending drug must be looked into, else further workup must be pursued.

Clinical Features

Hyperprolactinemia can manifest clinically either due to effect of prolactin on lactation and reproductive function or due to the underlying etiology.

Hyperprolactinemia can cause galactorrhea. However, it may be only intermittent. It is seen in up to 80% of women, but is uncommon in men because it requires estrogen or progesterone priming of the breast tissue. Hence, it is also uncommon in postmenopausal females.

Hypogonadotropic hypogonadism as a consequence of prolactin excess manifests differently in males and females. The characteristic triad of amenorrhea, galactorrhea, and infertility points to prolactin excess. Amenorrhea can be primary or secondary. Mild levels of prolactin excess may cause just shortening of luteal phase. It can even lead to infertility. Males present with decreased libido, erectile dysfunction, and infertility. Hypogonadotropic features like decreased muscle mass and body hair may be present. There can be osteoporosis in both sexes.

If prolactinomas are the underlying cause, it can manifest as visual field abnormalities and headache. Other tumors especially if large and infiltrating, can cause hypopituitarism, cranial nerve palsies, pituitary apoplexy, seizures due to temporal lobe extension, CSF rhinorrhea or hydrocephalus.

Approach

Hyperprolactinemia is diagnosed when fasting serum prolactin levels are >20 ng/mL in males and >25 ng/mL in females. In evaluation of such a case, one needs to first rule out physiological and drugs as etiology before proceeding to further workup. The first step in workup for hyperprolactinemia would be to confirm by repeating serum prolactin value especially if it is borderline or after stopping the possible offending drugs.

Further evaluation includes eliciting history of pregnancy, drug intake, visual difficulty, headache, hypothyroidism, renal failure, cirrhosis, seizure, chest wall surgery or trauma, nonfasting sample, and vigorous exercise. Also, one must elicit history of galactorrhea and hypogonadism. Examination of the patient for galactorrhea, chest wall injury, signs of hypogonadism, hypothyroidism, and visual field charting should be carried out. Laboratory investigation like renal and liver function, TSH, IGF-1 and evaluation of other pituitary hormones as appropriate.

Measurement of serum prolactin may be fallacious in two situations. One is hook effect where very high levels of prolactin may be reported as normal as they saturate the detecting antibody used for the assay. This can be overcome by 1:100 dilution of the serum sample. Similarly, a patient with very high levels of serum prolactin may not have clinical abnormality. This may be due to macroprolactin, which are aggregates of prolactin with immunoglobulins. These may be elevated in renal failure. This artifact can be overcome by pretreatment of the sample with polyethylene glycol before the immunoassay.

The MRI of the head to rule out a mass lesion in pituitary or hypothalamus is frequently needed. Evaluation of other pituitary hormones may be needed if sellar mass lesion is found. If no lesion is found, it is labeled as idiopathic.

Treatment

Indication for treatment includes impending neurological symptoms due to large size of adenoma or symptoms of hypogonadism or galactorrhea. The treatment of hyperprolactinemia depends on etiology.

Medical management with dopamine agonists is the treatment of choice for prolactinomas. Bromocriptine and cabergoline are approved for the same. These act on D2 receptors on lactotrope and decrease prolactin secretion. They are highly effective in 80–90% cases in improving prolactin levels, size of prolactinoma, correcting menstrual irregularities. Bromocriptine is initiated in low doses 1.25 mg daily and can be increased to 2.5 mg thrice a day. Cabergoline is initiated at 0.25 mg weekly and can be increased to 0.25 mg twice a week or 0.5 mg once a week. Initial doses can cause significant first dose effect like nausea, hypotension, etc., and hence smaller doses should be taken with meals to surpass these. Bromocriptine can be given intravaginal if not tolerated orally. The other adverse effects include exacerbation of psychosis, valvular regurgitation, nasal stuffiness, peripheral vasospasm, etc. Valvular regurgitation is uncommon at doses used in management of hyperprolactinemia. In general, cabergoline is better tolerated than bromocriptine. Cardiac ultrasound is recommended every 2 year if patient is on >2 mg per week of cabergoline. Prolactin levels should be repeated after 4 weeks of starting treatment. If there is normalization of prolactin levels on initiation of dopamine agonists, then they need to be continued. If there is decrease in level, but still no normalization, then dose of the drug needs to be increased. One may switch from bromocriptine to cabergoline if there is no response to bromocriptine. The drugs may be discontinued if there is no evidence of adenoma for >2 years on MRI.

Some cases are resistant to action of dopamine agonists. These have decreased expression of dopamine receptor or may be less well differentiated. These may require surgery or radiation therapy for management. In patients with microadenomas who do not respond to dopamine agonists and have hypogonadism, replacement with estrogen or testosterone; or ovulation induction with clomiphene may be needed.

Surgery has a limited role in management of prolactinoma. It is more effective in microadenoma than macroadenoma. Recurrence after surgery is relatively high. Hence, surgery is limited to cases with resistance to dopamine agonist therapy or if the prolactinomas are large enough to cause mass effects in patients planning pregnancy. Surgery can be combined with prior dopamine agonists to decrease size of macroadenomas or with postsurgery radiotherapy for management of residual tumor.

Other causes of hyperprolactinemia should be managed accordingly, e.g., hypothyroidism needs to be corrected. Drug-induced hyperprolactinemia due to antipsychotics (dopamine antagonists) may be a bit challenging as it may not be possible to discontinue the offending drug. In such cases, adding dopamine agonist under careful supervision or switching to atypical anti-psychotics should be attempted.

In selected patients with macroadenomas who become pregnant on dopaminergic therapy and who have not had prior surgical or radiation therapy, bromocriptine or cabergoline is continued throughout the pregnancy, especially if the tumor is invasive or is abutting the optic chiasma. Surgical resection may even be necessary in some cases.

CONCLUSION

Hyperprolactinemia is a very common clinical problem and should be evaluated meticulously. Drugs are the most common cause and should be ruled out first. Persistent hyperprolactinemia merits MRI. Dopamine agonists are the drugs of choice in management of prolactinoma.

Acknowledgments

- Dr Saba Samad Memon was involved in writing the manuscript and managing the case.
- Dr Ashraf Ganie was involved in supervising the case management and in editing the manuscript.
- Dr Sudhir Bhimaniya was involved in radiological diagnosis and selection of images for the manuscript.
- Dr Hammadur Rahaman also reviewed the manuscript and provided inputs.

SUGGESTED READINGS

1. Huang W, Molitch ME. Evaluation and Management of Galactorrhea. Am Fam Physician. 2012;85(11):1073-80.
2. Majumdar A, Mangal NS. Hyperprolactinemia. J Hum Reprod Sci. 2013;6(3):168-75.
3. Melmed S, Casanueva FF, Hoffman AR, et al. Diagnosis and Treatment of Hyperprolactinemia: An Endocrine Society Clinical Practice Guideline. J Clin Endocrinol Metab. 2011;96(2):273-88.
4. Wang AT, Mullan RJ, Lane MA, et al. Treatment of hyperprolactinemia: a systematic review and meta-analysis. Syst Rev. 2012;1:33.

6

CHAPTER **Diabetes in Young**

Srinivasa P Munigoti

CLINICAL VIGNETTE

A 22-year-old recently graduated engineer presents with history of polydipsia and polyuria, tiredness, and significant weight loss. Patient has no significant past medical history and comes with a family history of his grandfather being diagnosed of diabetes in his late 70s. His blood pressure at the time of presentation to the clinic is noted to be 140/94 mm Hg. He is noted to have acanthosis nigricans and his body mass index (BMI) measures 33 kg/m^2. His fasting blood sugar is noted to be 265 mg/dL and 2 hours post-75 g glucose value being 394 mg/dL with glycosylated hemoglobin (HbA1c) value of 11%.

What is the likely diagnosis in this young gentleman, type 2 diabetes mellitus (T2DM) or latent autoimmune diabetes in adults (LADA) or maturity-onset diabetes of the young (MODY)? Does differentiating various forms of this diabetes alter his management? How should one proceed with treatment in this patient?

Diabetes in Young—What Could it be—LADA or Type 1 Diabetes Mellitus (T1DM) or T2DM?

The term "latent autoimmune diabetes in adults," abbreviated as LADA, is normally used to describe a subgroup of patients who present with phenotypic appearance at an age identified commonly with T2DM. But, these patients have markers of autoimmunity like in T1DM. Genetic studies have identified LADA to be associated with higher frequency with human leukocyte antigen (HLA)-DR3 (28%), DR4 (27%), and DR3/4 (22%) similar to that of T1DM. The strength of this association is observed to decline with age. Two smaller studies looking at similarities in HLA and MICA5.1 also supported the same association between LADA and T1DM.

Norwegian-based HUNT study, looking at phenotypic differences between individuals with antibody-positive LADA and T2DM, identified that in those without the need for insulin, markers of metabolic syndrome were equally prevalent and pronounced. Whereas in insulin-treated individuals of the same study group, patients with LADA were leaner (mean BMI 28.7 kg/m^2) than patients with T2DM (mean BMI 30.9 kg/m^2). This difference in their BMI, although was statistically significant, remained marginal in absolute sense. A variety of observational data from numerous studies support a similar view that although patients with LADA may remain slightly leaner compared to patients with T2DM, their shared phenotypic features continue to confound clear distinction between them. Thus, in metabolic terms, the distinction between T2DM mellitus (T2DM) and LADA is not always clinically apparent.

So, LADA shares autoimmune markers with T1DM and presents with a phenotype resembling that of T2DM.

LATENT AUTOIMMUNE DIABETES IN ADULTS— "DEFINITION" AND THE DIFFICULTIES

Given this understanding, the term LADA, coined by Tuomi et al., was originally intended to distinguish this entity from classic T1DM, where insulin is required from diagnosis and from T2DM, where insulin is not required at all or at least until some years after diagnosis.

The diagnosis of LADA is currently based on three criteria: (1) Adult age at onset of diabetes (the Immunology of Diabetes Society proposes 30 years of age as a cutoff) (2) Lack of a requirement for insulin for at least 6 months after diagnosis, and (3) The presence of circulating islet autoantibodies.

Although this criterion gives a sense of clarity to the term itself, various components pose practical challenges in their usage to define the entity in clinical practice. To start with, age as a primary criterion remains arbitrary. Prevalence of antibodies in younger adults than specified in definition criteria is well described in all the various intermediate forms of diabetes reducing its discriminant value.

Autoantibody-positive adults who get initially treated for a brief while with insulin and later shifted to other forms of treatment essentially excludes them from being labeled as LADA, even if they demonstrate rapid beta-cell failure at a later date re-establishing need for insulin within short time after the diagnosis. Acknowledging problem in using insulin treatment as a defining measure is important because the decision to start insulin is likely to be influenced by preconceptions, local clinical practice, and also as a precaution to minimize ketosis.

The UK Prospective Diabetes Study (UKPDS) demonstrated the utility of antibodies in the management of diabetes mellitus (DM). In this landmark study, during recruitment, diagnosis of T2DM was made clinically and was assumed true, based on absence of ketonuria. Study subjects were divided into intensive therapy with tight glycemic targets using sulfonylurea/insulin as need be and conventional therapy using diet alone and those who were obese were chosen for metformin therapy. Autoimmune antibodies were measured at the baseline before the start of therapy. Looking at the results of 1,870 people who were not randomized to insulin arm, 5.8% of patients had islet cell antibodies and 9.8% had glutamic acid decarboxylase (GAD) antibodies, whereas 3.9% had both. More than 50% of patients who had one of the antibodies needed insulin within 6 years of diagnosis and it rose to nearly 80%, if both antibodies were positive. In contrast, only 4.5% of patients who did not have antibodies needed insulin. Although at first glance, this data looks promising in the utility of antibodies in predicting need for insulin with a specificity of 94.6% but the sensitivity was lower, i.e., 37.9%. This means that about two-thirds of the patients who need insulin lacked GAD antibodies, thus the positive predictive value is very less.

We also need to remember that autoimmune markers change over time and, hence, patients who had positive earlier results may turn negative in later life and vice versa. Work from Kimpimäki et al. and Hampe et al. showed us that antibodies tend to disappear more commonly in children than in adults and islet cell antibodies do so more often than GAD antibodies.

Given age and no insulin use for 6 months postdiagnosis remaining elusive as deterministic traits and antibodies of unpredictable prognostic value, usefulness of current criteria of diagnosis of LADA to practicing clinicians remains of questionable value.

Does Differentiation between LADA and T2DM Change Clinical Management?

The UKPDS, yet again, seems to provide valuable insights. Randomization to various treatment strategies at diagnosis also made it a quasi-controlled trial for testing comparative clinical outcomes for LADA. The patients with autoimmune diabetes are more likely to need insulin early on, but the results showed that after 10 years the patients who were randomized initially to diet or sulfonylurea therapy did not have any difference in glucose-dependent outcomes from those initially randomized to insulin.

Given this, the clinical benefits of diagnosis of LADA leading up to earlier use of insulin remains unproven as opposed to careful monitoring and treatment of hyperglycemia without any diagnosis, but with progressively escalating therapy that may initially include oral hypoglycemic agents.

Although shared immune markers with T1DM raise a potential possibility of immunomodulatory treatment in early stages of disease in LADA, there is no scientific study so far that has proven such therapy in LADA and, hence, screening and diagnosis even at early stage carries no therapeutic value.

Diabetes in Young—MODY versus T2DM versus T2DM—Which One is it?

Maturity-onset diabetes of the young is a clinically heterogeneous group of genetic disorders with an autosomal dominant mode of inheritance, charac-terized by DM, and an onset usually before the age of 25 years. 1–2% of patients diagnosed with diabetes are estimated to have MODY. It is prudent to distinguish MODY from T1DM and T2DM not only for treatment, but also for screening and early intervention because first-degree relatives have a 50% probability of inheriting the same mutation (autosomal dominant), which confer >95% lifetime risk of developing diabetes.

The expression of these genes is in the beta-cells and mutation of any of them leads to beta-cell dysfunction and DM. There are 14 known subtypes of MODY and mutations in three genes [*HNF1A*, hepatocyte nuclear factor 4A (*HNF4A*), and *GCK*] account for about 95% of all MODY cases. MODY 2 is associated with mutations in the gene that encodes the glycolytic enzyme glucokinase and the other five mutations are identified in genes that encode transcription factors: *HNF4A*, and *HNF1A*, identified with MODY 1 and 3, respectively, insulin promoter factor-1 (IPF-1) with MODY 4, *HNF1B* with MODY 5, and neurogenic differentiation 1 (NEUROD1), also known as beta-cell E-box transactivator 2 (BETA2), leading to MODY 6. The other uncommon genes are *ABCC8, KCNJ11, INS, PDX1, NEUROD1, CEL, KLF11, PAX4, BLK, and APPL1.*

Table 1 below illustrates clinical features associated with mutations in genes that cause MODY.

Despite an array of different mutations, three among this group of disorders seem particularly common and, hence, highly relevant to clinical practice. These most commonly present as mild, asymptomatic hyperglycemia in children, and young adults with a strong and multigenerational family history of diabetes, given its autosomal dominant pattern of inheritance. Due to mild nature of illness, the diagnosis may not be made until adulthood.

MODY 2

This is known to occur as a result of mutations in glucokinase gene and hyperglycemia in this group of persons appears to result from a reduction in the sensitivity of beta-cells to glucose as well as a defect in postprandial glycogen synthesis in the liver. Several mutations numbering >100 have been identified so far in the glucokinase gene. Most of these heterozygous mutations unlike homogenous ones are associated with a milder form of nonprogressive hyperglycemia that can be treated with diet alone. In most carriers who are affected, glycemic intolerance that includes mild fasting hyperglycemia and/or impaired glucose tolerance may be recognized at a very young age soon after birth and nearly half of the women who carry these mutations may develop gestational diabetes. Insulin therapy is rarely required in about 2% of cases. The complications of diabetes are rare in this form of MODY and as patients have mild hyperglycemia, these patients need no treatment. Patients may present with gestational diabetes will need treatment to minimize the impact on the obstetric outcomes.

TABLE 1: Clinical features associated with mutations in genes that cause maturity-onset diabetes of the young (MODY).

Genes	Relative prevalence	Other clinical features
HNF1A	Common (30–70% of MODY)	Low renal threshold for glycosuria; marked sensitivity to sulfonylureas
HNF4A	5–10% of MODY	Renal threshold for glycosuria is normal; marked responsiveness to sulfonylureas; neonatal hyperinsulinemia may be presenting feature and hypoglycemia may be associated with macrosomia; low concentrations of high-density lipoprotein/high concentrations of low-density lipoprotein
GCK	Common (30–70% of MODY)	Patients may have mild fasting hyperglycemia throughout life and are often detected during screening; small incremental glucose rise after carbohydrate load
HNF1B	5–10% of MODY	Genitourinary tract malformations (especially renal cysts and other renal developmental abnormalities); pancreatic atrophy and exocrine insufficiency
IPF1	Very rare	Pancreatic agenesis in homozygotes/compound heterozygotes
INS	Rare: <1% of MODY	More usually associated with neonatal diabetes
CEL	Very rare: Fewer than five families reported	Exocrine pancreatic dysfunction
NEUROD1	Very rare	Fewer than five families reported
KCNJ11	Rare: <1% of MODY	More usually associated with neonatal diabetes; sulfonylurea responsive
ABCC8	Rare: <1% of MODY	More usually associated with neonatal diabetes; sulfonylurea responsive

Source: Reproduced with permission from Thanabalasingham G, Owen KR. Diagnosis and management of maturity onset diabetes of the young (MODY). BMJ. 2011;343:d6044.

MODY 1 and MODY 3

HNF-α gene mutations are common and well-recognized form of MODY. The pathophysiologic mechanisms due to mutations in the HNF4A gene (MODY 1) and HNF1A gene (MODY 3) are very similar. The HNF4A regulates the expression of HNF1A. Deficiency of HNF4A is noted to be significant enough to lead to progressive hyperglycemia secondary to relative inability of beta-cells to overcompensate with time. Like persons with glucokinase mutations, this group of patients also may present with a mild form of diabetes. The plasma glucose concentrations 2 hours after glucose administration are much higher in patients with glucokinase mutations. More often than not, patients with mutations in HNF1A- or HNF4A-related MODY respond well to sulfonylureas. But their hyperglycemia is observed to increase over time, resulting in the need for insulin in a substantial proportion of these patients. Nearly 30–40% of patients with this form of mutations need insulin unlike 2% in those with MODY 2.

TABLE 2: Various clinical characteristics that distinguish these forms of diabetes from type 1 diabetes mellitus and type 2 diabetes mellitus.

Features	Type 1 diabetes mellitus	Type 2 diabetes mellitus	GCK-maturity-onset diabetes of the young (MODY)	HNF1A/4A-MODY
Typical age of diagnosis (years)	10–30	>25	Present from birth; presents at any age	15–45
Diabetic ketoacidosis	Common	Rare	Rare	Rare
Insulin dependent	Yes	No	No	No
Parental history of diabetes	<15%	>50% in young-onset type 2 diabetes mellitus	If tested, one parent usually has impaired fasting glycemia (may not be previously known)	60–90%[‡]
Obesity	Uncommon	Common	Uncommon	Uncommon
Insulin resistance	Uncommon	Common	Uncommon	Uncommon
Presence of β-cell antibodies	>90%	Negative	Rare	Rare
C-peptide concentrations	Undetectable/low	Normal/high	Normal	Normal
Optimal first-line treatment	Insulin	Metformin	None	Sulfonylurea

[‡] Maturity-onset diabetes of the young should, hence, be suspected when a patient who appears to have early-onset T2DM with a strong family history of multigenerational diabetes. Although higher BMI does not exclude the diagnosis, patients with MODY tend to be leaner than patients with T2DM.

Source: Reproduced with permission from Thanabalasingham G, Owen KR. Diagnosis and management of maturity onset diabetes of the young (MODY). BMJ. 2011;343:d6044.

Table 2 above illustrates various clinical characteristics that distinguish these forms of diabetes from T1DM and T2DM.

MODY should also be suspected when relatively young lean diabetic patient masquerading T1DM presents with negative autoantibodies and a measurable C-peptide level.

Is MODY Identified in India?

In India, genetic screening of monogenic diabetes has gained even more importance as T2DM is well established to present at least a decade earlier than it does in Caucasians. So, diagnosis of gene mutations leading up to MODY has significant implications. Clinical studies by Mohan and team earlier reported on the high prevalence of MODY (4.8%) in Chennai.

The "Centre for Advanced Research (CAR) in genomics" formed with joint collaboration of the Madras Diabetes Research Foundation (MDRF) and the Indian Council of Medical Research (ICMR) conducted project entitled "Study of Genes related to MODY and Early-onset Diabetes" aimed at determining the prevalence of MODY in different regions of India and to screen the known *MODY* genes for mutation and to examine their association with the causation of the disease status in Indians. Various studies done as part of this project identified MODY 1, 2, 3, 4, 5, 9, 11, and 12 genes in Indians. Project team also identified a novel *HNF1A* gene mutation Arg263His that was found to cosegregate with diabetes in a family in South India, causing the disease. Sulfonylurea-responsive mutations such as *KCNJ11* and *ABCC8* genes were also identified in number of screened patients leading to change in treatment for children from insulin treatment to oral drugs.

Does Differentiating Monogenic Diabetes (MODY) Help in the Management?

Identifying MODY 2 in children and young adults would certainly avoid unnecessary treatment for mild hyperglycemia. Similarly, diagnosis of MODY 1 and 3 in children and young adults would reduce use of unnecessary insulin at a young age, as many of them will respond to simple oral hypoglycemic agents. Identifying these mutations should also lead to selective screening of family members, thus helping in their early diagnosis and treatment.

CONCLUSION

Latent autoimmune diabetes in adults remains immunologically similar in presentation to T1DM. Poor positive predictive value of antibodies and phenotypic similarities make it difficult to identify it as a separate entity in clinical practice. Keen follow-up of glycemic response or lack of it to oral hypoglycemic agents remain the only pragmatic approach to manage this group of patients.

Maturity-onset diabetes of the young, as a well-proven genetic form of diabetes, is as much prevalent in India and distinguishing it by subjecting high probability group of diabetic patients such as children and very young adults with a strong family history to genetic screening that may have huge implications not only for screening but also for early and correct treatment.

CLINICAL CASE

Going back to our clinical case, our patient presented with phenotypic markers of T2DM (acanthosis nigricans and obesity). He also had significant hyperglycemia with no family pedigree pointing toward MODY making monogenic diabetes an unlikely diagnosis. Given poor utility of autoimmune antibodies (despite potential positivity) in distinguishing LADA from T2DM as discussed, trial of oral hypoglycemic agents, with careful follow-up and insulin initiation at the earliest need, should achieve similar results.

SUGGESTED READINGS

1. Antosik K, Borowiec M. Genetic Factors of Diabetes. Arch Immunol Ther Exp (Warsz). 2016;64(Suppl 1):157-60.

2. Broome DT, Pantalone KM, Kashyap SR, Philipson LH. Approach to the Patient with MODY-Monogenic Diabetes. J Clin Endocrinol Metab. 2021;106(1):237-50.

3. Byrne MM, Sturis J, Clément K, Vionnet N, Pueyo ME, Stoffel M, et al. Insulin secretory abnormalities in subjects with hyperglycemia due to glucokinase mutations. J Clin Invest. 1994;93:1120-30.

4. Horton V, Stratton I, Bottazzo GF, Shattock M, Mackay I, Zimmet P, et al. Genetic heterogeneity of autoimmune diabetes: age at presentation in adults is influenced by HLA DRB1 and DQB1 genotypes (UKPDS 43). UK Prospective Diabetes Study (UKPDS) Group. Diabetologia. 1999;42:608-16.

5. Hosszúfalusi N, Vatay A, Rajczy K, Prohászka Z, Pozsonyi E, Horváth L, et al. Similar genetic features and different islet cell autoantibody pattern of latent autoimmune diabetes in adults (LADA) compared with adult-onset type 1 diabetes with rapid progression. Diabetes Care. 2003;26:452-7.

6. Malecki MT, Jhala US, Antonellis A, Fields L, Doria A, Orban T, et al. Mutations in NEUROD1 are associated with the development of type 2 diabetes mellitus. Nat Genet. 1999;23:323-8.

7. Molven A, Njølstad PR. Role of molecular genetics in transforming diagnosis of diabetes mellitus. Expert Rev Mol Diagn. 2011;11(3):313-20.

8. Ramachandran A, Mohan V, Snehalatha C, Bharani G, Chinnikrishnudu M, Mohan R, Viswanathan M. Clinical features of diabetes in the young as seen at a diabetes centre in south India. Diabetes Res Clin Pract. 1988;4(2):117-25.

9. Todd JN, Srinivasan S, Pollin TI. Advances in the Genetics of Youth-Onset Type 2 Diabetes. Curr Diab Rep. 2018;18(8):57.

10. Velho G, Petersen KF, Perseghin G, Hwang JH, Rothman DL, Pueyo ME, et al. Impaired hepatic glycogen synthesis in glucokinase-deficient (MODY-2) subjects. J Clin Invest. 1996;98:1755-61.

7
CHAPTER

Rhinocerebral Mucormycosis in a Post-transplant Diabetes Mellitus Patient after Renal Transplant

Monika Goyal, Chandar Mohan Batra, Ashok Sarin, Ameet Kishore

INTRODUCTION

Mucormycosis is a rare, invasive fungal infection caused by fungus of order zygomycetes and includes family *Rhizopus, Mucor, Absidia, Apophysomyces,* and *Cunninghamella.* This disease predominantly occurs in uncontrolled diabetic patients especially in the setting of diabetic ketoacidosis and immunocompromised patients, though, studies show 20% infections occur in immunocompetent patients. Mucormycosis can be of five subtypes depending upon primary site of involvement, of which rhino-cerebral mucormycosis is overall most common type, while pulmonary is most common type in patients with solid organ transplant. *Rhizopus arrhizus* is the most common species worldwide while *Apophysomyces variabilis* is most common species in Asian countries. Treatment needs multidisciplinary approach with an attempt to make early diagnosis, early initiation of antifungal therapy, reversal of underlying risk factors, and surgical debridement with aggressive conservative approach. We present a case of 48-year-old patient with hypertension, primary hypothyroidism, pulmonary tuberculosis, chronic kidney disease, and post renal transplant, who was on triple immunosuppression [wysolone, mycophenolate mofetil (MMF), and tacrolimus].

CASE HISTORY

A 48-year-old male, a case of chronic kidney disease, post renal transplant patient on triple immunosuppression tablet wysolone 20 mg, tablet MMF, and tablet tacrolimus, was brought to the emergency department of Apollo hospital with complaints of fever on and off since 1 month, polyuria, and polydipsia since 10 days, breathlessness since 4 days, and altered sensorium since 3 days. Patient was initially admitted to another hospital for initial management where he was diagnosed with post-transplant diabetes mellitus (PTDM). Patient was a known case of chronic kidney disease and had undergone renal transplant in December, 2018 and was on triple immunosuppression with steroids, MMF, and tacrolimus since then, doing well till recently with no evidence of graft dysfunction. Patient also had history of pulmonary tuberculosis and had received modified antitubercular treatment (ATT). Patient also had hypertension and primary hypothyroidism; he on was on regular treatment. On examination, patient was febrile, tongue was dry and coated, had tachycardia, blood pressure was 110/70 mm Hg, no pedal edema, RBS by glucometer was high (>600 mg/dL). Patient had bilateral basal crepitations, drowsy not following verbal command, extraocular movements were normal, both pupils were normal and reactive to light, moving all four limb on deep painful stimulus. Laboratory investigations were done which showed anemia (Hb 9 g/dL), leukopenia (TLC 3,000/mm^3), increased blood urea 132 mg/dL and serum creatinine 3.6 mg/dL, high uric acid 10.7 mg/dL, and high sodium 162 mEq/L. ABG showed metabolic acidosis with pH of 7.29, pCO$_2$ 21, HCO$_3$ 10. Urine ketones were negative. Chest X-ray was suggestive of prominent bronchovascular marking. Blood and urine cultures were sent. A diagnosis of lower respiratory tract infection was made with PTDM with nonketotic hyperosmolar coma and acute kidney injury. Patient was started on antibiotics (targocid and meropenem), intravenous fluids and insulin infusion to control sugars; hydrocortisone was continued while other immunosuppressants were stopped. Further management was done on the lines of nonketotic hyperosmolar coma. By day 3, patient was out of nonketotic hyperosmolar coma, sugars were controlled, vitals had started stabilizing, consciousness improved, now patient had started following simple verbal commands. But on day 4, patient's condition started deteriorating suddenly. Patient was in shock, was requiring two vasopressor to maintain blood pressure of 96/66 mm Hg, and was intubated on pressure support ventilation to maintain a saturation of 98%. Patient was unconscious, not responding to deep pain stimulus, right eye proptosis was present, with chemosis and complete ophthalmoplegia in right eye. NCT showed opacity in the right maxillary sinus (**Fig. 1**). A diagnosis of mucormycosis was suspected with or without cavernous sinus thrombosis. Patient was promptly started on liposomal amphotericin B in the dose of 5 mg/kg along with posaconazole 400 mg BD. MRI could not be done since patient was not stable. ENT surgeon did urgent functional endoscopic sinus surgery (FESS) which showed presence of necrotic tissue, growing fungal hyphae on lateral aspect, and candida on the medial aspect of nasal cavity (**Figs. 2A to C and 3**). Samples were taken for direct microscopy, culture, and histopathological examination (HPE) which confirmed the diagnosis. The KOH mount of the nasal sample showed aseptate branching fungus at right angles suggestive of mucormycosis (**Fig. 4**). The biopsy tissue showed subcutaneous edema and aseptate branching fungal growth suggestive of mucormycosis (**Fig. 5**). The fungal culture confirmed growth of mucormycosis. Unfortunately, the patient's condition deteriorated further, he went into severe septic shock, finally succumbed to infection late that day in the evening.

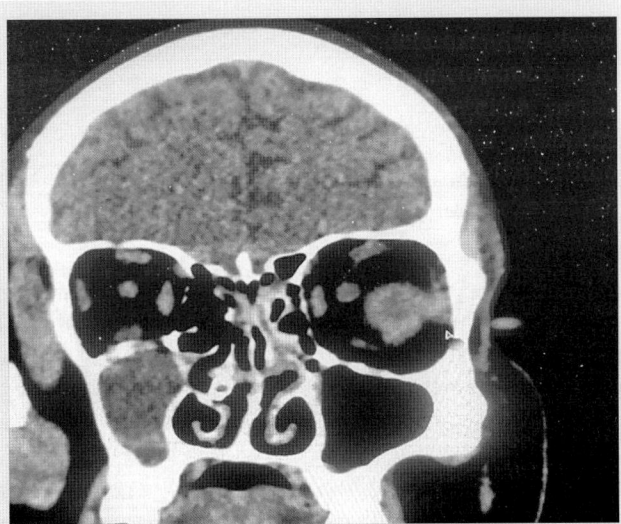

FIG. 1: NCCT of brain and sinus coronal view showing opacity in right maxillary sinus.

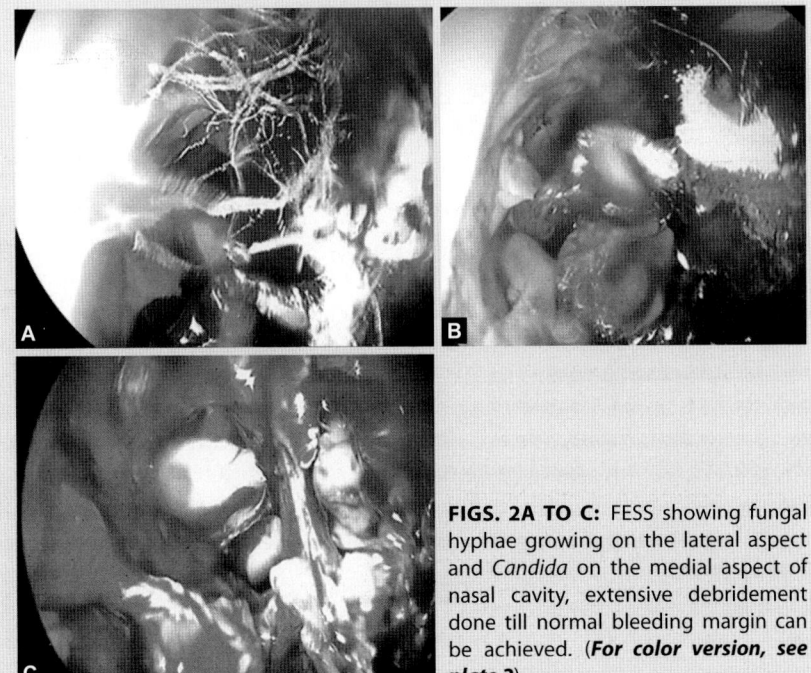

FIGS. 2A TO C: FESS showing fungal hyphae growing on the lateral aspect and *Candida* on the medial aspect of nasal cavity, extensive debridement done till normal bleeding margin can be achieved. (***For color version, see plate 2***)

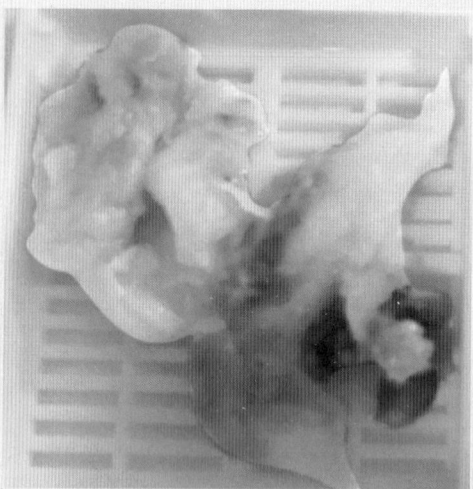

FIG. 3: Gross examination of tissue obtained on functional endoscopic sinus surgery showing dead, necrotic tissue. (*For color version, see plate 2*)

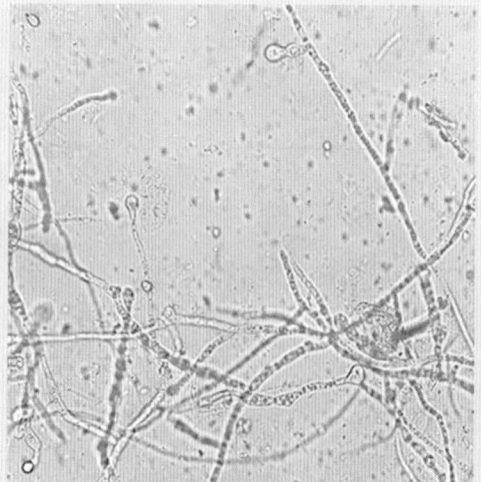

FIG. 4: KOH mount of the nasal sample showing aseptate branching fungus at right angle suggestive of mucormycosis and few budding yeast cell. (*For color version, see plate 3*)

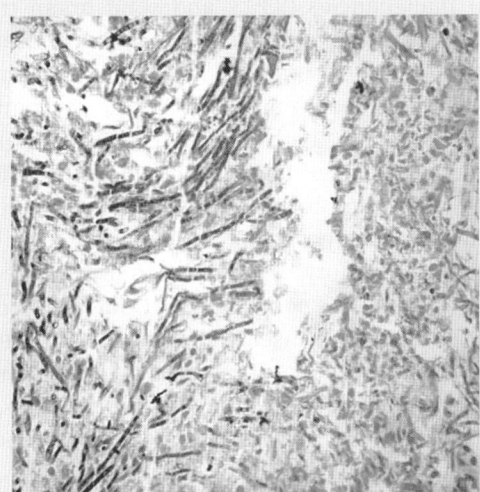

FIG. 5: Histopathological examination of biopsy tissue showing columnar epithelium, subcutaneous edema, aseptate, branching fungal growth suggestive of mucormycosis. (*For color version, see plate 3*)

DISCUSSION

Zygomycosis is rare, invasive fungal infection caused by function of order mucorales and includes family *Rhizopus, Mucor, Absidia, Apophysomyces,* and *Cunninghamella.* The fungus causes infection mainly by gaining entry into human body via respiratory tract or skin, though, less commonly can also enter via gastrointestinal (GI) tract. They invade tissue and causes arterial thrombosis and ischemic necrosis of the tissue.

Morphologically, they are characterized by presence of broad aseptate hyphae and formation of zygospores. *R. arrhizus* is the predominant identified species followed by *Rhizopus* microspores whereas *Apophysomyces variabilis* is emerging as an important species in south Asian population.

Mucormycosis can be of five types depending upon its site and location, i.e., rhinocerebral mucormycosis, pulmonary, cutaneous, GI or disseminated. Rhinocerebral mucormycosis is the most common type especially in the setting of uncontrolled diabetes. Mucormycosis Sino-nasal or Sino-orbital disease with involvement of brain accounts for 66% of mucormycosis in diabetic patient; however, in solid organ transplant recipient patient pulmonary infection is the most predominant site accounting for 39% of patients.

Multiple risk factor predispose to mucormycosis including diabetes and diabetic ketoacidosis being the most common (35%) cause followed by hematological malignancies (33%), and solid organ transplant (13%), persistent neutropenia, deferoxamine therapy, illicit use of intravenous drugs, prophylaxis with voriconazole and echinocandins, and breach of cutaneous or mucous membrane barrier due to trauma, burns, and surgical wounds. Our patient had multiple predisposing risk factors, i.e., immunosuppression, use of steroids, PTDM, and acidosis. Identifying these risk factors is very important as an early step to reverse them to improve prognosis. Recent meta-analysis done by Jeong W et al. suggested even though 33% patient had history of corticosteroids, its role as a risk factor for mucormycosis could not be confirmed and warrants further evaluation. Until recently believed to be a disease of immunocompromised patients, two meta-analysis done at different time periods documented ~19% of the mucormycosis cases occurred in immunocompetent hosts, in which most common type was cutaneous followed by rhinocerebral mucormycosis.

Clinical presentation of mucormycosis depends on the site of infection and can affect patient of any age, race, sex, and occupation. Majority presents as subacute presentation while some present with rapid progressing disease, chronic infections are rare. Patient with rhinocerebral mucormycosis present with fever, sinusitis, rhinitis, granular or purulent discharge, nasal ulceration, epistaxis, facial pain and swelling, orbital cellulitis, diplopia, complete ophthalmoplegia like in our case, hemiplegia or stroke, and decreased mental function. The disease is usually unilateral but can become bilateral. Pulmonary infection is seen most commonly in severe neutropenic patients, on chemotherapy, leukemia, patients on long-term antibiotics, post hematopoietic stem cell transplants patients especially those with graft versus host disease. It present mainly with dyspnea, cough, chest pain, fever, and hemoptysis. Predisposing factors for cutaneous mucormycosis are trauma are burns, persistent macerated skin, insulin injection site, and catheter insertion site. They develop necrotizing fasciitis which spreads locally rapidly, may progress to involve subcutaneous tissue and muscle rarely may go for dissemination. GI mucormycosis is seen in malnourished patients, especially, malnourished children mainly as necrotizing enterocolitis. Studies show that patients with solid organ transplants are at higher risk of developing GI mucormycosis presenting with nonspecific complains of pain in abdomen, abdominal bloating or rarely hematochezia. Dissemination is characterized by infection at two or more contagious site. About 23% patients may develop disseminated disease. About 9–26% patients of solid organ transplant have risk of disseminated disease with maximum risk in liver transplant patient 26–55%. About 50% of patients with pulmonary, 38% with GI infection, and 20% patient with cutaneous infection suffered from dissemination.

Diagnosis is challenging because of nonspecific symptoms and rarity of disease. Imaging plays an important role and may help in early diagnosis. A study of patients with rhinocerebral mucormycosis found that 100% patients show soft tissue mucosal thickening on CT scan with mild enhancement seen in 70% of patients, 40% of patients show evidence of bone erosion, rarefactions, and permeative destruction. In MRI, 100% patients show lesion as hypodensity on T1 weight images with variable intensity of T2 images and variable contrast enhancement. In case of pulmonary mucormycosis, radiologically lesion seen in decreasing order of frequency are consolidation, mass, cavitation, and wedge-shaped infarct. Features suggestive of mucormycosis are presence of sinusitis, multiple nodules on CT (>10), and pleural effusion. Reverse halo is an early sign and most likely to be seen in mucormycosis. It is seen in 20–90% patients (**Fig. 6A** and **B**).

Even though imaging may give an early supportive evidence of mucormycosis, in the background of relevant clinical scenario, demonstration of mucormycosis is mandatory to make either a proven or probable mucormycosis as defined by European Organization for Research and Treatment of Cancer/Mycoses Study Group. To make a definitive diagnosis of mucormycosis, a combination of a positive mucorales culture and microscopic evidence is mandatory. This is possible only in quarter of cases. In remaining cases, diagnoses could reasonably be made on the basis of a combination of clinical features and the identification of nonseptate, right-angled branching hyphae. The diagnostic utility of HPE or direct microscopy of biopsied tissue is clearly evident. In a meta-analysis, HPE of tissue has contributed in diagnosis of mucormycosis in 97% of cases. Besides the presence of broad, nonseptate hyphae, branching at wide angle with evidence of tissue invasion remains a criterion for classifying mucormycosis as proven infection and also helps in differentiating from more common aspergillosis that has septate hyphae. Likewise, mucorales can be grown in culture which helps in morphological evaluation, identifying species and genus, to run an antifungal susceptibility test, though it is positive only in

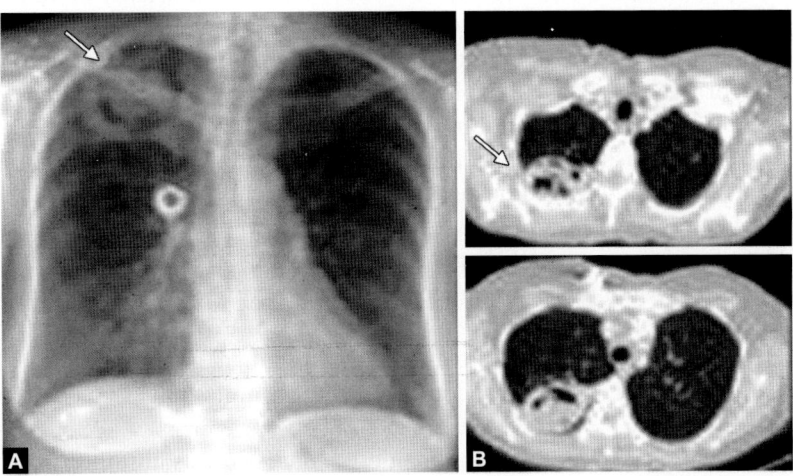

FIGS. 6A AND B: Chest X-ray of patient with pulmonary mucormycosis showing reverse halo sign.

53% of cases. The various mediums that can be used to grow mucorales are brain heart infusion broth, potato dextrose agar, and sabouraud dextrose agar with gentamycin and polymyxin B without cycloheximide. New modern molecular-based methods are available that help in early identification of species including less common pathogenic species, though its clinical utility is limited because of lack of standardization and clinical validation technique. Large scale studies are required to know their role as primary diagnostic modality in the diagnosis of mucormycosis.

The successful treatment of mucormycosis requires four steps, i.e., early diagnosis, early initiation of polyene therapy, reversal of underlying risk factors, and early surgical debridement. Study show starting polyene therapy within 5 days after diagnosis of mucormycosis was associated with improvement in survival, compared with initiation of polyene therapy at ≥6 days after diagnosis (83% vs. 49% survival). Amphotericin B is the primary line of treatment of mucormycosis. Liposomal amphotericin B appears to be least toxic and has maximum central system penetration. No guidelines are available on the use of primary combination therapy due to lack of prospective study but on the basis of few studies done on diabetic rats amphotericin B with echinocandins appear to be reasonable strategy as an initial combination therapy. Though combination therapy of amphotericin with posaconazole is commonly used therapy but is not FDA approved since the minimum inhibitory concentration (MIC) of drug required for antifungal activity cannot be achieved at approved therapeutic dose of drug. Deferasirox with amphotericin was recommended earlier until Deferasirox-AmBisome Therapy for Mucormycosis (DEFEAT Mucor) study was released. It was first randomized trial for any treatment of mucormycosis with one arm receiving treatment with amphotericin b and deferasirox while other arm receiving amphotericin B with placebo. The results found 45% mortality at 30 days and 82% mortality at 90 days in deferasirox treated arm. Thus, suggesting that deferasirox cannot be recommended as part of an initial combination regimen for the treatment of mucormycosis. Posaconazole is quite a popular salvage therapy in patient intolerant to amphotericin B therapy or if it is contraindicated due to other reasons. Other adjunctive therapies have been used in few patients including granulocyte transfusion, granulocyte colony stimulating factor (GCSF), granulocyte-macrophage colony-stimulating factor (GM-CSF), interferon (IFN)-gamma improving phagocytic function, hyperbaric oxygen (100% oxygen at atmospheric pressure for 90 minutes twice a day to provide adequate oxygen level to improve killing capacity of neutrophils, alleviates acidosis thus inhibiting fungal growth). Others like lovastatin and VT-1161 (otesaconazole) that inhibits fungal CYP51 have also been used.

Early surgical treatment is considered necessary as thrombosis and resulting tissue necrosis during mucormycosis can result in poor penetration of antifungal agents to the site of infection. Retrospective review support the concept of "aggressive conservative" approach in which intraoperative frozen sections are used to delineate the margins of infected tissues and uninvolved tissues are spared from debridement whenever possible. Surgery was found to be an independent variable for favorable outcomes in patients with mucormycosis.

Prognosis is usually bad even with early initiation treatment. A prospective study done in north showed the overall mortality rate of mucormycosis ranges from 38 to 56.5%. The primary site of infection play an important role in determining the outcome. Marked increase in mortality is seen when dissemination occurs with reports of 100% mortality with central nervous system (CNS) dissemination in some studies. Mortality has been reported from 33 to 60% from isolated pulmonary infection that increase to 95% when disseminated, 85–100% for GI infection, 10–17% for cutaneous infection (94% when disseminated), and 31–93.3% for rhinocerebral infection (98% when disseminated to CNS). The highest treatment outcomes were achieved with *Rhizopus* species followed by *Mucor* and mycocladus (68%, 59%, and 50% respectively). Unfortunately, despite timely diagnosis, early institution of antifungal drugs and early surgical intervention we could not save our patient.

CONCLUSION

Mucormycosis is a rare fungal infection mainly affecting immunocompromised or uncontrolled diabetic patient, though increasing incidences are being seen in immunocompetent. Diagnosis is based on high index of suspicion along with appropriate imaging finding, HPE, microscopy, and using new molecular diagnostic test. Early initiation of combination of medical and surgical line of treatment improves the survival. Over all prognosis continue to remain poor especially in disseminated disease.

SUGGESTED READINGS

1. Bala K, Chander J, Handa U, et al. A prospective study of mucormycosis in north India: experience from a tertiary care hospital. Med Mycol. 2015;53(3):248-57.
2. Chakrabarti A, Singh R. Mucormycosis in India: unique features. Mycoses. 2014;57 (Suppl 3):85-90.
3. De Pauw B, Walsh TJ, Donnelly JP, et al. Revised definitions of invasive fungal disease from the European Organization for Research and Treatment of Cancer/Invasive Fungal Infections Cooperative Group, National Institute of Allergy and Infectious Diseases Mycoses Study Group (EORTC/MSG) Consensus Group. Clin Infect Dis. 2008;46(12):1813-21.
4. Goldstein EJ, Spellberg B, Walsh TJ, et al. Recent advances in the management of mucormycosis: from bench to bedside. Clin Infect Dis. 2009;48(12):1743-51.
5. Jeong W, Keighley C, Wolfe R, et al. The epidemiology and clinical manifestations of mucormycosis: a systematic review and meta-analysis of case reports. Clin Microbiol Infect. 2019;25(1):26-34.
6. Prakash H, Chakrabarti A. Global epidemiology of mucormycosis. J Fungi (Basel). 2019; 5(1):26.

7. Singh N, Aguado JM, Bonatti H, et al. Zygomycosis in solid organ transplant recipients: a prospective, matched case-control study to assess risks for disease and outcome. J Infect Dis. 2009;200(6):1002-11.

8. Spellberg B, Ibrahim AS, Chin-Hong PV, et al. The Deferasirox–AmBisome Therapy for Mucormycosis (DEFEAT Mucor) study: a randomized, double-blinded, placebo-controlled trial. J Antimicrob Chemother. 2012;67(3):715-22.

9. Therakathu J, Prabhu S, Irodi A, et al. Imaging features of rhinocerebral mucormycosis: A study of 43 patients. The Egyptian Journal of Radiology and Nuclear Medicine. 2018;49(2):447-52.

8
CHAPTER

Thalassemia and Endocrine Disorders

Kranti Khadilkar, Shilpa Prabhu, Subramaniam Kannan

CASE 1

A 14-year-old girl diagnosed as thalassemia major at 4 months of age and on monthly blood transfusions, she was referred to the endocrine clinic for short stature and delayed puberty. Her weight was 24 kg (<3rd percentile) and height was 120 cm (<3rd percentile) with target height range of 164 ± 6.5 cm (50th percentile). She had typical hemolytic facies with generalized hyperpigmentation and prepubertal sexual maturity rating (SMR) without any breast or pubic/axillary hair development. Her bone age was 10 years and investigations showed a normal serum calcium of 8.5 mg/dL and a high thyroid-stimulating hormone (TSH) of 20 µIU/mL (normal: 0.4–4.5 µIU/mL) and a thyroxine (T4) of 4.5 µg/dL (normal: 4.2–11.5 µg/dL) suggestive of primary hypothyroidism. Patient was started on 50 µg of levothyroxine daily. After a month of T4 and rendering her euthyroid growth, gonadotropin axes were tested. Laboratories revealed age- and sex-matched low insulin-like growth factor 1 (IGF-1) level of 40 ng/mL (normal: 95–618 ng/mL) and undetectable gonadotropins [follicle-stimulating hormone (FSH) of <0.4 mIU/mL and luteinizing hormone (LH) <0.3 mIU/mL]. Her growth hormone (GH) studies showed a low peak GH level (3 ng/mL) on clonidine stimulation test. She was started on GH therapy and subsequently on estrogen and progesterone. This case exemplifies the several endocrine issues occurring in thalassemia major—short stature (GH deficiency), delayed puberty (hypogonadotropic hypogonadism), and primary hypothyroidism.

CASE 2

An 11-year-old boy with beta-thalassemia major, who has been receiving monthly blood transfusions from 6 months of age and started on deferoxamine therapy since 9 years of age, presented with polyuria, polydipsia, and weight loss of 15 days duration. Random blood glucose was 527 mg/dL at his hometown and was referred to our clinic. His height was 137 cm (25–50th percentile) and weight was 25 kg (10th percentile) with body mass index (BMI) of 13.3 kg/m^2. Clinical examination revealed hepatosplenomegaly and pre-pubertal genitalia. His fasting glucose was of 230 mg/dL and postprandial glucose was of 440 mg/dL. His transaminases were elevated at alanine aminotransferase (ALT) of 124 IU/L (normal: 24–68 IU/L) and aspartate aminotransferase (AST) of 88 IU/L (normal: 10–36 IU/L). His serology tested positive for hepatitis C. His TSH was 1.12 µIU/mL, free T4 was 0.98 ng/dL (normal: 0.6–1.8 ng/dL), corrected serum calcium was 8.3 mg/dL (normal: 8.5–10 mg/dL), serum 25-hydroxyvitamin D was 25.69 ng/mL, and parathyroid hormone (PTH) was 2.1 pg/mL (normal: 10–75 pg/mL). A noncontrast CT scan of the abdomen is shown in **Figure 1**. CT scan of the abdomen revealed a high attenuation values of liver and pancreas (80–90 HU) (**Fig. 1**) consistent with iron overload. His serum ferritin was 2,076 ng/mL (normal: 22–322 ng/mL). Ferriscan MRI T2 for the heart was 19.4 ms suggesting mild iron deposition. Patient was initiated on insulin infusion and later transitioned to split-mixed insulin regimen. At follow-up in 6 months, patient's sugars were controlled on approximately 2 units/kg/day of insulin with fasting glucose of 130 mg/dL and postprandial glucose of 160 mg/dL. Patient's iron chelation therapy was intensified.

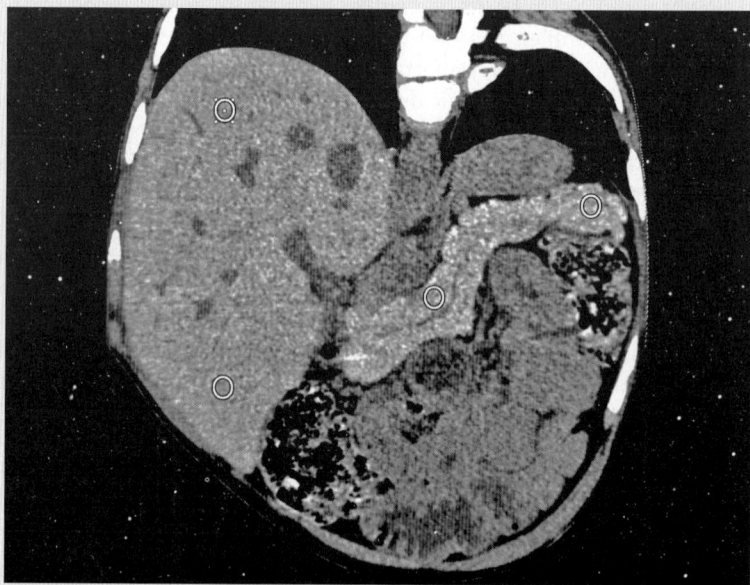

FIG. 1: Panoramic reconstructions of coronal sections of noncontrast CT scan of the abdomen showing a high attenuation of the liver and the pancreas consistent with iron overload (circles).

CASE 3

A 24-year-old female presented with right upper quadrant abdominal pain for duration of 2 weeks with intermittent nausea. She was evaluated and on ultrasonography (USG), there was a large right adrenal mass. Computed tomography (CT) examination demonstrated a 5 × 6 cm heterogeneous right adrenal mass, which showed uneven contrast enhancement and a moderate mass effect. There was an inferior displacement and deformity of the right kidney (**Fig. 2**). The mass was well defined, heterogeneous with hypodense areas, and showed minimal enhancement with contrast. The left adrenal gland was normal. She did not have any hypotension or features suggestive of adrenal insufficiency. Her blood pressure was normal at 110/70 mm Hg. Her liver was palpable 2 cm below the right costal margin and her spleen tip was palpable. Her hemoglobin (Hb) was 6.3 g/dL and mean corpuscular volume (MCV) was 64 fL. Rest of the blood counts were normal. Hb electrophoresis revealed a double heterozygous HbE-thalassemia (HbE: 72%; HbF: 15%; and HbA2: 7.7%). 24 hours urine metanephrines and catecholamines were normal. CT-guided biopsy of the adrenal mass showed adrenocortical tissue along with hematopoietic elements, mostly erythroid precursors in various stages of maturation with a few myeloid and megakaryocytic lineage cells (**Fig. 3**) and no adipose tissue. The final diagnosis was adrenal extramedullary hematopoiesis. She is being managed conservatively with blood transfusions and hydroxyurea and we plan to repeat imaging in 6 months.

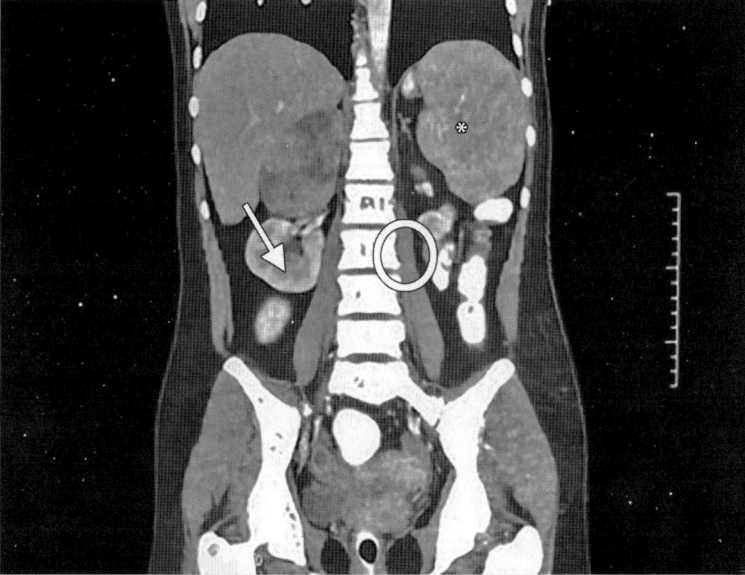

FIG. 2: Postcontrast CT scan (sagittal) shows a heterogeneous well-defined right adrenal mass with minimal contrast enhancement displacing the right kidney inferiorly (arrow). Also noted is a normal left adrenal gland (circle) and splenomegaly (asterisk).

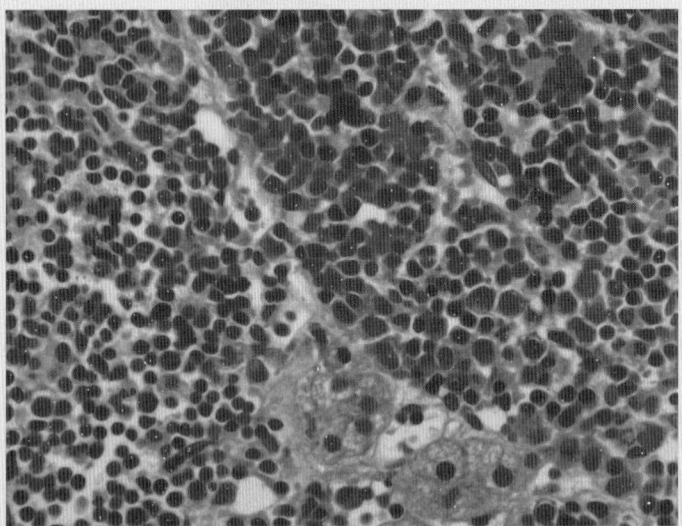

FIG. 3: Hematoxylin and eosin (H&E) stain at magnification (40×) shows adrenocortical tissue along with hematopoietic elements. It mostly shows erythroid precursors in various stages of maturation. Also seen are a few myeloid and megakaryocytic lineage cells. No adipose tissue is seen. This was consistent with a diagnosis of extramedullary hematopoiesis. (***For color version, see plate 4***)

CASE 4

A 15-year-old boy with beta-thalassemia with manifestation of iron overload, including diabetes, short stature, and delayed puberty, underwent open laparotomy and splenectomy. Postoperatively, patient developed severe hypocalcemic tetany in the third postoperative day requiring intravenous calcium infusions. Corrected calcium at the time of symptoms was 6.2 mg/dL. Other laboratories included a phosphorus of 8 mg/dL (normal: 3.5–5.5 mg/dL), magnesium level of 1.1 mg/dL (normal: 1.7–2.3 mg/dL), 25-hydroxyvitamin D level of 12 ng/mL (normal: >20 ng/mL), and intact PTH of 4 pg/mL (normal: 10–75 pg/mL). This was consistent with hypoparathyroidism, which typically gets manifest after a stressful event, generous intravenous saline infusions, infections, etc. Patient was started on oral calcium, active vitamin D (calcitriol), magnesium, and was slowly weaned off the intravenous calcium infusions.

INTRODUCTION

Thalassemia major is a genetic disorder of Hb synthesis resulting in severe anemia requiring lifelong blood transfusions. The combination of transfusion and chelation therapy has dramatically extended the life expectancy of thalassemic patients, but it is complicated by iron overload resulting in a high incidence of endocrine abnormalities in children and young adults.

Types of endocrinopathies seen in thalassemia include short stature, delayed puberty, hypothyroidism, hypoparathyroidism, diabetes mellitus (DM), osteoporosis, and hypoadrenalism.

PATHOPHYSIOLOGY OF ENDOCRINOPATHY IN THALASSEMIA

Multiple transfusions and anemia resulting in increased absorption from gut contribute to iron overload in especially those tissues that harbor high levels of transferrin receptors such as the endocrine glands. The nontransferrin bound iron (NTBI), which is the free circulating form, generates reactive oxygen species leading to lipid peroxidation in the cells. It also inhibits antioxidant defenses such as superoxide dismutase causing oxidative damage to cells. Cytotoxicity is further augmented by chelators such as deferroxamine and chronic anemia and tissue hypoxia.

GROWTH IN THALASSEMIA

Poor growth and short stature are the most common endocrinopathies observed in thalassemia. Poor growth is multifactorial and seen in both undertransfused as well as well-transfused patients. Under transfusion, chronic anemia and subsequent hypoxia interfere with the growth plate resulting in poor growth. Iron overload and poor chelation protocols cause growth retardation through many possible mechanisms such as anterior pituitary somatotroph damage with poor GH secretion and impaired GH response to growth hormone-releasing hormone (GHRH). Iron overload, especially in the liver, results in abnormal GH receptors and reduced IGF-1 and insulin-like growth factor-binding protein 3 (IGFBP-3). Deferroxamine, one of the commonly used chelating agents, along with chelation of iron also chelates zinc, causes toxic effects on chondrocytes in the growth plate resulting in metaphyseal dysplasia.

The growth failure usually manifests after first decade and predominantly affects the sitting height because of poor growth of the vertebral bodies (platyspondyly). Another important contributing factor to poor final height is associated unrecognized endocrinopathies such as hypothyroidism and hypogonadism as well as complications of iron overload such as liver disorders, diabetes, and malnutrition.

Children with height 2 standard deviation (SD) below the mean height for age, sex, and midparental height, or growth velocity consistently below 25th percentile, should undergo testing for GH deficiency. The levels of IGF-1 and IGFBP-3, however, should be viewed cautiously in the background of liver dysfunction and malnutrition. One-third have frank GH deficiency and this group is benefitted with GH therapy, though the response is poor as compared to the other conditions such as Turner syndrome. Remaining, generally, have an attenuated peak response to provocation GH testing and some may also have a component of GH resistance. Such group of patients generally responds poorly to GH therapy.

Correction of anemia and malnutrition, calcium, zinc, and vitamin D supplementation, correction of other associated endocrinopathies such as hypothyroidism and hypogonadism as well as appropriate chelation therapy are essential for maximum growth potential.

PUBERTAL DELAY

Gonadotropins of the anterior pituitary are sensitive to the effects of iron overload and oxidative damage than the gonads; hence, secondary hypogonadism is more common than primary hypogonadism.

A mixed hypogonadism (primary + secondary) is also a well-known occurrence in thalassemia. Common presentation is a delayed or arrested puberty in both males and females commonly accompanied by short stature and other features of poor chelation. Hypogonadism leads to poor quality of life as well as a poor peak bone mass acquisition resulting in osteoporosis. It is important to screen the patients for hypogonadism and adequately treat them with sex hormone replacements. Sex hormone replacement therapy, starting with low doses and building up slowly, should be started at the appropriate age for pubertal induction, so that pubertal gain in height, adequate muscle mass, and peak bone mass is appropriately achieved.

DIABETES MELLITUS

Iron overload and resulting oxidative damage result in progressive beta-cell damage and insulin-dependent DM. Though some studies have also shown a component of insulin resistance, the mechanism is still unclear and use of insulin sensitizers is not studied. The presentation is rarely explosive such as type 1 diabetics, but generally more insidious with osmotic symptoms, poor growth, and pubertal delay. Hence, routine surveillance with blood glucose levels is advisable beyond first decade or earlier, if symptomatic. Diagnosis is based on the standard biochemical criteria; however, glycosylated hemoglobin (HbA1c) is not reliable for monitoring glycemic control due to presence of hemoglobinopathy. Treatment is with insulin and higher than expected dose requirement is to be expected with insulin resistance at the liver.

HYPOTHYROIDISM

Thyroid can be affected either as primary hypothyroidism (subclinical or overt) or rarely as secondary hypothyroidism (pituitary). As the onset and progression are gradual, it requires regular surveillance for early diagnosis. Early diagnosis and appropriate treatment have important beneficial effects in the general well-being, bone health and final height, and pubertal outcomes.

Annual TSH and T4 are recommended from 9 years of age or earlier, if symptomatic. Mild and overt hypothyroidism requires treatment whereas benefit of treating subclinical hypothyroidism should be based on the individual case scenario.

HYPOPARATHYROIDISM

Chronic iron overload results in parathyroid dysfunction presenting as overt hypocalcemia in 3–4% of patients, especially in the second decade. Subclinical parathyroid dysfunction with biochemical disturbances is, however, said to present in almost all patients with thalassemia major. Hypocalcemia has adverse consequences in terms of increased morbidity and poor quality of life. Hence, regular annual surveillance for the same should be ideally done in all thalassemia patients beyond the first decade or earlier, if symptomatic. The diagnosis is based on low serum calcium, high phosphate, and low PTH levels. Treatment should be started immediately with oral calcium (1 g of calcium/day) and calcitriol (0.25–1.5 µg/day), with frequent monitoring of serum and urine calcium levels. Tetany, seizures, or cardiac failure due to severe hypocalcaemia requires immediate intravenous (IV) administration of calcium.

OSTEOPOROSIS

Osteopenia and osteoporosis, especially of the hip and spine, are almost universally present in adolescent thalassemia patients. Basic pathology is poor peak bone mass acquisition resulting from multifactorial causes: Bone marrow expansion due to ineffective erythropoiesis, vitamin D deficiency, chronic liver disease, untreated hypothyroidism, DM, and hypogonadism. Diagnosis is established early by bone mineral density estimation by using dual-energy X-ray absorptiometry (DXA) studies with appropriate corrections for short stature.

Improved nutrition with dietary calcium and vitamin D supplementation, regular physical activity, and sex hormone replacement at the appropriate age, where necessary, can help prevent or halt the progress of osteoporosis. In established osteoporosis or presence of evidence of fragility fractures, bisphosphonate therapy is beneficial.

ADRENAL DISORDERS

Adrenal failure can be of primary or secondary (pituitary) in origin with biochemical hypocortisolemia commonly seen. However, adrenal crisis is rarely observed. Iron deposition in the adrenal gland can result in delayed or attenuated adrenarche along with subclinical hypocortisolemia as well as subclinical mineralocorticoid deficiency. Secondary adrenal insufficiency, resulting due to impaired pituitary function, may be seen distinguished from primary by affliction of only the cortisol axis. Early symptoms such as tiredness, weight loss, and muscle weakness could mimic those of chronic anemia. Diagnosis is established by a low basal (8 AM) cortisol and low adrenocorticotropic hormone (ACTH)-stimulated cortisol (<18 µg/dL, 60 min after 250 µg ACTH IV). Generally, in absence of overt insufficiency, only stress cover of steroids is required in thalassemia patients. A rare presentation could be a large adrenal mass representing an uncommon site for extramedullary erythropoiesis similar to the common sites such as liver and spleen. The mass could cause early satiety, pain, or may even result in rupture and, hence, may require removal.

The International Network on Endocrine Complications in Thalassemia (I-CET) position statement suggests following annual endocrine screening:
- This should be started from the age of 9 years or earlier, if clinically indicated
- Serum TSH and free T4
- Serum calcium, ionized calcium, inorganic phosphate, magnesium, and alkaline phosphatase
- Luteinizing hormone, FSH, and sex steroids in the pubertal age group
- Fasting glucose/insulin semiannually
- Calculate annual growth velocity (GV), BMI, and upper/lower segment ratio. GV below 25th percentile or height SD below third percentile or 2 SD below the mean height for age and sex and midparental height advise provocative GH testing
- Serum or hair zinc (in selected cases)
- Bone age (X-ray of wrist and hand)
- Radiographs of tibia and spine should be evaluated in patients with body disproportion to exclude the presence of platyspondylosis or metaphyseal cartilaginous dysplasia changes.

USE OF DEFERASIROX FOR PREVENTION OF ENDOCRINE COMPLICATIONS

The frequency of endocrine complications seen before the deferasirox treatment was 83% but while receiving deferasirox treatment, it was 25.8% ($p < 0.05$). Both existing endocrine abnormalities were reduced and recent developed problems were less likely with long-term deferasirox treatment in thalassemia patients.

CONCLUSION

Endocrine dysfunction is an unavoidable consequence of multiple transfusions and longer lifespan in patients with thalassemia. Multidisciplinary approach with joint clinics involving hematologists and endocrinologists, regular surveillance, early treatment, and frequent follow-up would help mitigate this issue.

SUGGESTED READINGS

1. Bajwa H, Basit H. Thalassemia. In: StatPearls [Internet]. Treasure Island (FL): StatPearls Publishing; 2021.
2. Bilgin BK, Yozgat AK, Isik P, Çulha V, Kacar D, Kara A, et al. The effect of deferasirox on endocrine complications in children with thalassemia. Pediatr Hematol Oncol. 2020;37: 455-64.
3. De Sanctis V, Soliman AT, Elsedfy H, Skordis N, Kattamis C, Angastiniotis M, et al. Growth and endocrine disorders in thalassemia: the International Network on Endocrine Complications in Thalassemia (I-CET) position statement and guidelines. Indian J Endocrinol Metab. 2013;17:8-18.
4. Galaris D, Pantopoulos K. Oxidative stress and iron homeostasis: mechanistic and health aspects. Crit Rev Clin Lab Sci. 2008;45:1-23.
5. Gulati R, Bhatia V, Agarwal SS. Early onset endocrine abnormalities in beta thalassemia major in a developing country. J Pediatr Endocrinol Metab. 2000;13:651-6.
6. Karimi M, Zarei T, Haghpanah S, Azarkeivan A, Kattamis C, Ladis V, et al. Evaluation of endocrine complications in beta-thalassemia intermedia (β-TI): a cross-sectional multicenter study. Endocrine. 2020;69:220-7.
7. Raiola G, Galati MC, De Sanctis V, Nicoletti MC, Pintor C, De Simone M, et al. Growth and puberty in thalassemia major. J Pediatr Endocrinol Metab. 2003;16:259-66.

9

CHAPTER **Myxedema Coma**

Justin Easow Sam, Pramila Kalra

INTRODUCTION

Myxedema coma is a rare but life threatening condition which occurs due to severe deficit of thyroid hormones. It can be precipitated by various factors like infections, hypothermia, cerebrovascular accidents, congestive heart failure and GI bleed. Low intracellular T3 is the basic underlying pathology in myxedema crisis. There are diagnostic scoring available for myxedema coma diagnosis. The basic principles of management includes intensive care treatment with correction of hypotension, hypothermia and aggressive management of precipitating factors and steroid supplementation. The thyroid hormone replacement should be started through intravenous route if available else 500 µg of oral loading dose of levothyroxine may be the next best option to be given at the earliest. The mortality in myxedema coma is very high and patient education about prevention is the best approach.

CASE HISTORY

A 60-year-old female patient is admitted to the accident and emergency department. She comes with complaints of drowsiness of 7 days' duration, reduction of motor coordination, and slight mental confusion. She also has history of fever 1 week back.

At admission, in the emergency room, the patient is somnolent but arousable. On examination, the pulse rate is 50/min, regular, all peripheral pulses are palpable. A blood pressure of 130/90 mm Hg, axillary temperature of 95°F, and pulse oximetry of 95% with no supplementation of oxygen are recorded. The peripheries are very cold to touch, with a capillary refill of >4 seconds. She is obeying verbal commands with a score in the Glasgow Coma Scale of 13 (2/5/6). There is no goiter or neck stiffness.

Other remarkable features are dry skin, macroglossia, puffy eyelids, thick lips, nonpitting edema over both legs. Neurological examination reveals sluggish deep tendon reflexes. The patient's lungs on auscultation are bilaterally clear and cardiac examination shows a regular rate and rhythm without murmurs, gallops, or rubs. The patient's abdomen is soft without signs of guarding, tenderness, or rebound tenderness.

The patient's laboratory values are as follows: Hemoglobin 11.8 g/dL, white blood cell (WBC) count 6,000/µL (86% neutrophils), serum sodium 121 mEq/L, serum potassium 4.2 mEq/L, serum chloride 87 mEq/L, blood urea nitrogen (BUN) 1.3 mg/dL, serum creatinine 0.6 mg/dL, glucose 104 mg/dL, alanine aminotransferase (ALT) 113 U/L, aspartate aminotransferase (AST) 74 U/L, serum albumin 3.3 g/dL, creatinine kinase (CK) 499 IU/L, serum creatine kinase 14,664 IU/L CK-MB 21.4 ng/mL, troponin-I <0.02 ng/mL, lactate 1.2 mM/L, and urine red blood cells (RBCs) 1–4/hpf.

Thyroid-stimulating hormone (TSH) is 227 mU/L, FT4 (free T4) <3 pmol/L, cortisol 10.7 ug/dL, and capillary blood glucose 54 mg/dL.

The 12-lead ECG (electrocardiography) shows sinus bradycardia, a chest X-ray shows left basal atelectasis, and possibly a small pleural effusion.

Transthoracic echocardiography shows no pericardial effusion, left ventricular systolic function moderately impaired, and right ventricular systolic function severely impaired. Abdominal X-ray reveals distended bowel loops indicating ileus.

DISCUSSION

Diagnosis, Causes, and Differential Diagnoses

Myxedema coma is a rare but life-threatening condition which occurs due to a severe deficit in the thyroid hormones resulting in the collapse of the metabolism.

Myxedema may be the first presentation of patients with undiagnosed hypothyroidism. Myxedema coma can be a result of any of the well-known causes of primary hypothyroidism, e.g., autoimmune thyroiditis and postsurgical hypothyroidism. Secondary hypothyroidism due to pituitary failure can also be a causative factor.

The precipitating factors are hypothermia, infections, cerebrovascular accidents, congestive heart failure, gastrointestinal (GI) bleeding, and trauma. Drugs such as anesthetics, sedatives, tranquilizers, narcotics, amiodarone, and lithium carbonate have also been implicated. Metabolic disturbances such as hypoglycemia, hyponatremia, hypoxemia, hypercapnia, acidosis, and hypercalcemia exacerbate myxedema coma.

Hashimoto encephalopathy, sepsis, and accidental hypothermia are the differential diagnosis of myxedema coma.

Epidemiology

Case series and case reports from the western world indicate an incidence of 0.22 cases per million per year. Approximately 5% had hypothalamic or pituitary disease as a cause of hypothyroidism. Analysis from a national in-hospital database in Japan showed an estimated incidence of 1.08 cases per million people per year in Japan.

In a study done by Dutta et al. which included 23 patients with myxedema coma, 39% of them had hypothyroidism detected only at the time of crisis; 17% had central hypothyroidism. Sepsis was the most common precipitating factor and significant proportion of patients (61%) had defaulted on their thyroid replacement therapy.

Etiopathogenesis

Low intracellular T3 due to hypothyroidism is the basic underlying pathology in myxedema crisis. Normal body core temperature is preserved in compensated hypothyroidism because of neurovascular adaptations which include chronic peripheral vasoconstriction, mild diastolic hypertension, and diminished blood volume. The diastolic hypertension is secondary to increased peripheral vascular resistance that occurs in hypothyroidism due to lack of the vasodilatory effect of T3 on the smooth muscle of the vasculature.

Low intracellular T3 also leads to depressed cardiac functions due to decreased inotropism and chronotropism with vasoconstriction.

Further decrease in blood volume (e.g., secondary to GI bleeding or use of diuretics) disrupts this precarious balance, which homeostatic mechanisms are no longer able to restore.

In the decompensated state, low cardiac output and hypotension lead to cardiogenic shock not responsive to vasopressors without thyroid hormone replacement. Decreased central nervous system (CNS) sensitivity to hypoxia and hypercapnia leads to respiratory failure exacerbated by intercurrent pulmonary infection and pneumonitis. Water retention and hyponatremia occur secondary to decreased glomerular filtration rate (GFR) (due to decreased renal perfusion resulting from decreased cardiac output), decreased volume delivery to distal nephron, and excess vasopressin.

Decreased gluconeogenesis, precipitating factors such as sepsis, and concomitant adrenal insufficiency may contribute to hypoglycemia.

Most patients with myxedema coma have normal serum cortisol concentrations, but adrenocorticotropic hormone (ACTH) and cortisol responses to stress may be slightly impaired. Factors such as decreased cerebral blood flow in addition to generalized depression of cerebral function, hypoglycemia, hypoxemia, and hyponatremia can precipitate focal or generalized seizures and worsen the level of consciousness.

Sedative, analgesic, antidepressant, hypnotic, antipsychotic, and anesthetic drugs are incriminated as precipitating or exacerbating myxedema coma because of their ability to depress respiration, particularly in hospitalized patients.

Clinical Features

The typical patient is an elderly woman presenting during cold weather. Past history of antecedent thyroid disease, thyroid hormone therapy that was discontinued for no apparent reason or radioiodine therapy is suggestive of pre-existing thyroid disease. Examination of the neck may reveal a surgical scar and no palpable thyroid tissue or goiter. Presence of orbitopathy is a subtle clue to underlying Graves' disease treated with radioiodine or surgery.

Characteristic features of severe hypothyroidism such as dry skin, sparse hair, hoarse voice, periorbital edema and nonpitting edema of hands and feet, macroglossia and delayed deep tendon reflexes, and moderate-to-profound hypothermia may be present.

Whatever the precipitating cause, the course is that of lethargy followed by stupor and then coma, associated with respiratory failure and hypothermia. This is hastened by administration of precipitating drugs that depress respiration and other brain functions.

Hypothermia is present in three-fourths of patients and will generally be the first clinical clue to diagnosis. The diagnosis also needs to be considered seriously in an unconscious patient with an infection who does not have fever. Patients having core temperatures below 90°F have the poorest prognosis. Hypoglycemia can exacerbate the hypothermia.

Cardiovascular manifestations include bradycardia, hypotension, cardiomegaly, low cardiac output pericardial effusion, cardiogenic shock bundle branch blocks, arrhythmias, and nonspecific ECG findings. Schenck et al. reported a patient with severe hypothyroidism who presented with presyncope, prolongation of QT interval, and polymorphic VT (torsades de pointes) which reversed with thyroid hormone supplementation.

Neurological manifestations are lethargy, confusion, obtundation, coma, seizures, poor cognitive function, depression, and psychosis.

Respiratory system features include hypoxia, hypercapnia, myxedema of larynx, pleural effusion, and pneumonia.

Renal features include fluid retention, anasarca, hyponatremia, and bladder atony. GI system manifestations are anorexia and nausea, abdominal pain, constipation paralytic ileus, toxic megacolon and gastric atony, neurogenic oropharyngeal dysphagia, and pneumonia (precipitating factor).

Coexisting adrenal insufficiency is associated with hypotension, hypoglycemia, hyponatremia, hyperkalemia, and azotemia.

Metabolic complications include hypoglycemia, hypothermia with urine sodium normal or increased, and urine osmolality greater than serum osmolality.

Precautions Need to be Taken When the Temperature is Checked

Mercury thermometers may underestimate the degree of hypothermia if mercury column is not lowered to well below normal before patient's temperature is measured. They also do not record below 94°F and hypothermia may be underestimated. Electronic thermometers are preferred as they record temperature over a much wider range.

Recent Case Reports of Rare Clinical Manifestations of Myxedema Coma

Rare cardiac presentations include sudden cardiac arrest, thoracentesis-reverting cardiac tamponade with large pleural effusion. Myxedema coma with concomitant nonconvulsive seizure and neuroleptic malignant syndrome are uncommon neurological presentations. Impending myxedema coma has also been reported as the initial presentation of lung cancer.

Diagnosis of myxedema coma may be complicated by renal failure. Myxedema coma has also been observed in the setting of hyperglycemic hyperosmolar state. Myxedema coma due to Hashimoto thyroiditis has also been a rare presentation of failure to thrive in infancy.

Diagnostic Tests and Available Scoring Systems

The presence of three key diagnostic features can suggest a diagnosis of myxedema coma which is as follows:
1. *Altered mental status*: From disorientation and lethargy to psychosis and coma
2. *Defective thermoregulation*: Hypothermia or the absence of fever despite an infectious disease
3. *Precipitating event*: Cold exposure, infection, drugs (diuretics, sedatives, and tranquilizers), trauma, stroke, heart failure, and GI bleeding

Hypotension, bradycardia, hyponatremia, hypoglycemia, and hypoventilation are often present as well.

There are no conclusive diagnostic tests available. The diagnosis is initially based upon the history, physical examination, and exclusion of other causes of coma and should be considered in any patient with coma or depressed mental status that also has hypothermia, bradycardia, and/or hypercapnia.

Presently, there are two scoring systems available at present (**Tables 1** and **2**).

Principles of Management

The principles of management are as follows:
- Intensive care treatment with ventilator support, central venous pressure (CVP) monitoring, and pulmonary capillary wedge pressure, if feasible in patients with cardiac disease.
- Appropriate fluid management and correction of hypotension and dyselectrolytemia.
- Aggressive management of precipitating factors and steroid supplementation, if required.
- Thyroid hormone replacement.

TABLE 1: Diagnostic scoring system for myxedema coma.

Thermoregulatory dysfunction (temperature, °C)		Cardiovascular dysfunction	
>35	0	**Bradycardia**	
32–35	10	Absent	0
<32	20	50–59	10
Central nervous system effects		40–49	20
Absent	0	<40	30
Somnolent/lethargic	10	Other ECG changes	10
Obtunded	15	Pericardial/pleural effusions	10
Stupor	20	Pulmonary edema	15
Coma/seizures	30	Cardiomegaly	15
Gastrointestinal findings		Hypotension	20
Anorexia/abdominal pain/constipation	5	**Metabolic disturbances**	
Decreased intestinal motility	15	Hyponatremia	10
Paralytic ileus	20	Hypoglycemia	10
Precipitating event		Hypoxemia	10
Absent	0	Hypercapnia	10
Present	10	Decrease in GFR	10

(ECG: electrocardiography; GFR: glomerular filtration rate)

Therapeutic Endpoints of Treatment

The therapeutic endpoints of treatment are as follows:
- Improved mental status
- Improved cardiac function
- Improved pulmonary function

Management of a Patient with Myxedema Coma

Myxedema coma is an endocrine emergency and should be treated aggressively.

Before specific therapy is initiated, blood should be drawn for measurements of serum thyrotropin (TSH), free T4, free T3, and cortisol. Other routine investigations which include complete blood count (CBC), S. creatinine, BUN, liver function, serum electrolytes, ECG, two-dimensional (2D) echo urine routine, chest X-ray, and blood and urine cultures should be done to identify precipitating factors and initiate treatment. An arterial blood gas (ABG) analysis must be done. An X-ray of abdomen will be helpful to rule out intestinal obstruction. Ideally, a short synacthen test should be performed to exclude adrenal insufficiency.

However, the emergency life-saving measures should not be delayed for the reports.

TABLE 2: Myxedema coma screening tool.

Criterion		Score
GCS		
• 0–10		• 4
• 11–13		• 3
• 14		• 2
• 15		• 0
TSH		
• >30 mU/L		• 2
• Between 15 and 30 mU/L		• 1
Low Free T4		1
Hypothermia		1
Bradycardia		1
Precipitating event		1
Total Scores	**Category**	**Recommendation**
8–10	Most likely	Proceed with treatment
5–7	Likely	Treat if there are no other plausible causes
<5	Unlikely	Consider other diagnosis

Free T4 <0.6 ng/dL.
Hypothermia: Body temperature <95°F measured on admission.
Bradycardia: Heart rate <60 bpm measured on admission.
Precipitating event: Burns, carbon monoxide retention, gastrointestinal hemorrhage, infection, sepsis, medications, stroke, surgery, trauma, etc.
(GCS: Glasgow Coma Scale; TSH: thyroid-stimulating hormone)

- *Ventilatory support:* The utmost priority is the management of airway and airway protection from aspiration in patients with a depressed consciousness level. Endotracheal intubation or tracheostomy with mechanical ventilation is to be done when required. ABG analysis is to be done for ensuring adequate oxygenation and correction of hypercapnia. Sedatives and other drug are to be avoided. Most patients require mechanical ventilatory support for 24–48 hours, especially those in whom hypoventilation was caused by drug-related respiratory depression and some may require it for several weeks.
- *Hypotension:* For fluid resuscitation, the choice is to be made between fluid supplementation for hypotension and fluid restriction for hypo-natremia. For hypotension, judicious administration of intravenous fluid initially with 5–10% glucose in half-normal sodium chloride is to be done. In case of hyponatremia, isotonic sodium chloride is preferred. In the presence of adrenal insufficiency, administration of hydrocortisone (100 mg intravenously every 8 h) is indicated. Vasopressors should be initiated, if required. Consider other causes such as sepsis, myocardial infarction (MI), pericardial effusion, and occult bleeding in cases of persistent hypotension.

- *Hyponatremia*: For mild hyponatremia (120–130 mEq/L), fluid restriction with replacement to cover daily losses taking care to supplement glucose, sodium, and potassium is to be done. However, if there is severe hyponatremia (<120), small amount of hypertonic saline (50–100 mL of 3% sodium chloride) is to be administered followed by an intravenous (IV) bolus of 40–120 mg of furosemide to promote water diuresis while continuing to closely monitor volume status so that serum sodium may be elevated by 3–4 mEq/L to tide over the immediate crisis. Though therapy with vasopressin antagonists is logical as some studies have shown increased vasopressin levels in myxedema, no reports of its use in this clinical circumstance are available and are presently not recommended.
- *Hypothermia*: Though thyroid hormone supplementation will restore body temperature to normal, its action is slow. Blankets are used to prevent heat loss and maintain temperature but provide minimal warming. Passive warming by keeping room temperature warm and use of standard blankets are advised.
- *Glucocorticoid therapy*: IV hydrocortisone in a dosage of 50–100 mg every 6–8 hours for several days is to be administered, after which it is tapered and discontinued on the basis of clinical response plans for further diagnostic evaluation.
- Thyroid hormone therapy (see below).

Special Precautions to be Taken During Management

Active warming with electric blankets should not be done as it causes vasodilatation and decreases peripheral vascular resistance further and thereby exacerbating hypotension.

Due to hypothermia, initial detection of infection is often complicated. As such, initiation of antibiotics is delayed or not given at all. It may justify providing antibiotic therapy to all patients with myxedema coma.

Intravenous glucocorticoids must be given to all patients before the initiation of thyroid hormone therapy as most patients with myxedema coma have normal serum cortisol concentrations, although their ACTH and cortisol responses to stress may be slightly impaired.

What should be Preferred—T4 or T3?

Because of the rarity of myxedema coma and paucity of studies of the effects of treatment, optimal therapy remains uncertain and several different approaches used and hence is the most controversial aspect of treatment. The main uncertainty is whether to administer T4 alone, with conversion to T3 being dependent on deiodinase activity in the patient, or to directly administer both T4 and T3. The secondary concerns are dose, frequency, and route of administration.

The high mortality of untreated myxedema coma and obvious need for attaining effective thyroid hormone concentrations in different tissues fairly rapidly should be balanced against the risks of high-dose thyroid hormone therapy such as atrial tachyarrhythmias or MI.

T4 alone provides a steady and smooth, but rather slow, onset of action with low-risk for adverse effects. T3 has a more rapid onset of action, but its serum (and probably tissue) concentrations fluctuate more between doses.

The American Thyroid Association (ATA) has recommended that the initial thyroid hormone replacement for myxedema coma should be IV levothyroxine (LT4). A loading dose of 200–400 μg of LT4 should be given, with lower doses given for smaller or older patients and those with a history of coronary artery disease (CAD) or arrhythmia. This is followed by a daily replacement dose of 1.6 μg/kg body weight (should be decreased to 75% when given IV). After the patient improves clinically, oral therapy or other enteral therapy can be used if the oral route cannot be employed.

Since T4 conversion to T3 may be decreased in patients with myxedema coma, the ATA states that IV liothyronine (LT3) may be given in addition to LT4. High doses are to be avoided due to increased mortality. Loading dose of 5–20 μg can be given, followed by maintenance dose of 2.5–10 μg every 8 hours, with lower doses for older patients and those with h/o CAD or arrhythmia. Therapy can continue until the patient is clearly recovering (e.g., until the patient regains consciousness and clinical parameters have improved). Significant clinical improvements are seen within 24 hours with T3, but the more rapid action of T3 is associated with a higher risk of adverse cardiovascular actions. High serum T3 concentrations during treatment with T3 alone are associated with fatal outcome in several patients.

What is to be Done if IV Levothyroxine is not Available?

Oral administration of T4 through Ryles tube is equally effective. The drawback is that gastric atony may prevent absorption and put the patient at risk for aspiration.

Dutta et al. compared 500 μg of an oral loading dose of T4 with 150 μg of maintenance dose orally and 200 μg of T4 IV followed by 100 μg T4 IV until they regained their vital functions and were able to take oral medications in patients with myxedema crisis and did not find any difference in outcome among patients.

Read et al. demonstrated that the rate of T4 absorption after oral adminis-tration of T4 through nasogastric tube was similar among hypothyroid and euthyroid (control) subjects. Arlot et al. reported on seven patients presenting with myxedema coma. Two of them received treatment with 1 mg intravenous T4 and rest received 0.5 mg LT4 orally on the first day; subsequent daily dose varied for each patient. As expected, plasma T4 and T3 of oral group increased more slowly than those of IV group. However, improvement in clinical outcome occurred within 24–72 hours in both groups.

So, an oral dose of 500 μg as a loading dose can be administered, since a dose of >500 μg/day of oral LT4 is associated with fatal outcome within 1 month of treatment according to one study.

A recent case report pointed out the effectiveness of a "split high-dose oral LT4 therapy" as an alternative treatment for myxedema coma and could be especially useful in elderly patients in light of the risk of adverse cardiovascular (CV) effects of single high-dose LT4 therapy. Oral administration of 0.2 mg LT4 every 8 hours in five consecutive doses (total dose of 1 mg) resulted in a significant restoration of depleted thyroid status and clinical improvement within 48 hours after treatment initiation.

Determining if a Pericardial Effusion in a Patient is Secondary to Hypothyroidism

Though pericardial effusion is rare in a patient with myxedema coma, a pericardial fluid analysis showing high cholesterol levels is suggestive that the effusion has occurred secondary to hypothyroidism.

Monitoring a Patient being Treated for Myxedema Coma

Thyroid hormones are to be measured every 1–2 days to ensure favorable trajectory in biochemical parameters. Though optimal levels for serum TSH and thyroid hormones are not well-defined, the failure of TSH to trend down or for thyroid hormone levels to improve can be considered as indications to increase LT4 therapy and/or add LT3 therapy. A high-serum T3 is an indication to decrease therapy.

Prognosis

Myxedema coma has a mortality rate of about 40%. Cases of myxedema coma usually occur in women with a significant mortality rate (25–60%), even when they are under proper treatment.

CONCLUSION

The best preventive approach is patient education. The mortality rate is about forty percent. The patients need to be monitored in intensive care and if IV levothyroxine is not available then high stat oral dose of levothyroxine should be administered immediately.

SUGGESTED READINGS

1. Arlot S, Debussche X, Lalau J-D, et al. Myxoedema coma: Response of thyroid hormones with oral and intravenous high-dose L-thyroxine treatment. Intensive Care Med. 1991;17(1):16-8.
2. Charoensri S, Sriphrapradang C, Nimitphong H. Split high-dose oral levothyroxine treatment as a successful therapy option in myxedema coma. Clin Case Rep. 2017;5(10):1706-11.
3. Chen YC, Cadnapaphornchai MA, Yang J, et al. Nonosmotic release of vasopressin and renal aquaporins in impaired urinary dilution in hypothyroidism. Am J Physiol Renal Physiol. 2005;289(4):F672-8.
4. Chiong YV, Bammerlin E, Mariash CN. Development of an objective tool for the diagnosis of myxedema coma. Transl Res. 2015;166(3):233-43.
5. Dutta P, Bhansali A, Masoodi S, et al. Predictors of outcome in myxoedema coma: a study from a tertiary care centre. Crit Care. 2008;12(1):R1.

6. Jonklaas J, Bianco AC, Bauer AJ, et al. Guidelines for the treatment of hypothyroidism: Prepared by the American Thyroid Association Task Force on thyroid hormone replacement. Thyroid. 2014;24(12):1670-751.

7. Ladenson PW, Goldenheim PD, Ridgway EC. Prediction and reversal of blunted ventilatory responsiveness in patients with hypothyroidism. Am J Med. 1988;84(5):877-83.

8. Mathew V, Misgar RA, Ghosh S, et al. Myxedema coma: a new look into an old crisis. J Thyroid Res. 2011;2011:1-7.

9. Ono Y, Ono S, Yasunaga H, et al. Clinical characteristics and outcomes of myxedema coma: Analysis of a national inpatient database in Japan. J Epidemiol. 2017;27(3):117-22.

10. Popoveniuc G, Chandra T, Sud A, et al. A diagnostic scoring system for myxedema coma. Endocr Pract. 2014;20(8):808-17.

11. Read DG, Hays MT, Hershman JM. Absorption of oral thyroxine in hypothyroid and normal man. J Clin Endocrinol Metab. 1970;30(6):798-9.

12. Reinhardt W, Mann K. Häufigkeit, klinisches Bild und Behandlung des hypothyreoten Komas. Med Klin. 1997;92(9):521-4.

13. Schenck JB, Rizvi AA, Lin T. Severe primary hypothyroidism manifesting with torsades de pointes. Am J Med Sci. 2006;331(3):154-6.

14. Wartofsky L. Myxedema coma. Endocrin Metab Clin North Am. 2006;35(4):687-98.

10

Thyroid-associated Orbitopathy

Veechika Reddy, Pramila Kalra

CASE 1

A 38-year-old female presents with 2 months history of significant weight loss, increased appetite, palpitations, sweating, tremulousness, loose stool, and heat intolerance. She also complains of grittiness, photophobia, gaze-evoked pain, and some change in the appearance of both the eyes about the same duration. There is no associated diplopia. Her eye symptoms have only a minor impact on her daily life. Her menstrual cycles are regular. She has no comorbidities or any family history of thyroid disorder. She is not on any medications. She is a nonsmoker.

On physical examination, she is alert and anxious. Temperature: 98.7°F, pulse rate (PR): 120 beats/min, blood pressure (BP): 120/50 mm Hg, respiratory rate (RR): 16 breaths/min, and weight: 52 kg. Her extremities are warm, moist, and she has fine tremors of the hands. There is a World Health Organization (WHO) grade II goiter with no nodularity on palpation.

On eye examination, lid retraction of about 1.5 mm is noted in both eyes. The exophthalmometric values in the both eyes are about 18 mm. Mild erythema of the conjunctive is seen. No chemosis, eyelid swelling, or erythema has been noted. Visual acuity, color vision, visual fields, and extraocular movements were normal. Fundus examination was normal. A clinical activity score of 2/7 has been recorded.

Her blood investigations and 99mTc scan of thyroid are suggestive of Graves' diseases (GDs).

Her thyroid-stimulating hormone (TSH): <0.001 µIU/mL, thyroxine (T4): 20 µg/dL, and triiodothyronine (T3): 350 ng/dL.

---

1. **What is thyroid-associated orbitopathy (TAO)?**

   Graves' ophthalmopathy (GO), thyroid eye disease (TED), or TAO is an immune-mediated inflammatory disorder that leads to expansion of the extraocular muscles and fat in the orbit. Up to 95% of thyroid-associated ophthalmopathy is seen in patients with GD. About 5% of patients with ophthalmopathy have primary hypothyroidism rather than GD (**Fig. 1**).

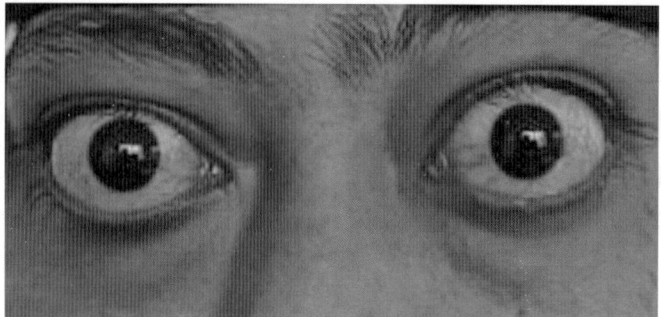

FIG. 1: Graves' orbitopathy. (***For color version, see plate 4***)

2. What is the epidemiology of GO?

Graves' ophthalmopathy is a relatively rare disease. The incidence of GO in general population in the United States has been reported as 16 women and 3 men per 100,000 population per year.

Graves' ophthalmopathy is clinically evident in about 40% of patients with GD; considering a prevalence of GD of 1% in general population, the prevalence of GO is about 0.4%. About two-thirds of all GO patients have mild GO. The overall prevalence of GO is estimated to be about 90/100,000 population (60/100,000 for mild GO and 30/100,000 for moderate-to-severe GO). Asians have lesser prevalence of GO (7.8%) compared to Caucasians (34%).

The age distribution has two peaks, one at 40–44 years and a later one at 60–64 years for women and 65–69 years for men.

The disease is more common in females with a female-to-male ratio of 9.3 in patients with mild orbitopathy, 3.2 in those with moderate orbitopathy, and 1.4 with severe orbitopathy. This indicates that male sex is a risk factor for developing severe ophthalmopathy.

The incidence of GO has been declining in the last few decades, probably related to a decline in the prevalence of smokers, to an earlier diagnosis and treatment of Graves' hyperthyroidism (facilitated by the introduction of sensitive TSH assays in the 1980s), and to a prudent use of 131I therapy.

3. What is the pathogenesis of GO?

Current evidence suggests an autoimmune pathogenesis with genetic and environmental influences. An autoantigen TSH receptor (TSHR) is shared between the thyroid and the orbit. It is expressed in the orbital fibroblasts, orbital fat, and extraocular muscle fibers at a higher level in patients with GO than normal subjects. The TSHR autoantibody in GD patient binds to the TSH in the orbital tissues eliciting an inflammatory response leading to infiltration by lymphocytes and macrophages. Not only TSHR, insulin-like growth factor-1 (IGF-1) receptor expression is also increased in orbital tissues in patients with GO, which may have a pathogenic role.

The expansion of orbital tissue is secondary to the deposition of hydrophilic glycosaminoglycans synthesized by the orbital fibroblasts in response to cytokines and increase in the orbital fat content secondary to differentiation of orbital fibroblasts into adipocytes. This stage of infiltration is followed by fibrosis. As orbit is a rigid cone, this edematous expansion leads to increased orbital pressure, proptosis, and dysfunction of affected muscles.

The clinical expression depends upon the site and severity of inflammatory response and the potential for forward displacement. If the orbital septum is lax, it leads to proptosis limited by the ability of the orbital muscle to stretch. If the septum is tight and the muscle is unable to stretch, it leads to increased orbital pressure and venous congestion leading to compression of optic nerve with minimal proptosis, an entity defined as concealed proptosis which is uncommon but has a high risk for optic neuropathy. Optic neuropathy commonly develops as a result of pressure from enlarged muscles on the optic nerve or the vessels that supply it.

Infiltration and fibrosis of extraocular muscles lead to restriction of eye movements, lid lag, and incomplete eye closure leading to sight-threatening corneal exposure. The most commonly affected muscles are inferior rectus followed by medial, superior, levator, lateral rectus, and oblique.

Acute inflammation may lead to erythema and swelling of the eyelids and conjunctivae, compounded by venous and lymphatic congestion.

4. What are the risk factors for the occurrence of GO?

Both genetic and environmental factors increase the susceptibility for GO. Advanced age, male sex, tobacco use, biochemically more severe hyperthyroidism, high TSHR antibodies, and 131I therapy have been identified as risk factors. Genetic factors include polymorphisms in HLA-DR3, HLA-DRB1, CTLA4, PTPN22, CD40, interleukin (IL)-2RA, FCRL3, IL-23R, IL-3, IL-21, and IL-23 are associated with GO. Recent studies found single nucleotide polymorphism (SNP) in ARID5B and NRXN3 that are associated with fat deposition in orbital tissue. By far, smoking is the most important risk factor compared to other genetic factors.

5. What is the natural history of GO?

Graves' ophthalmopathy can precede or follow thyrotoxicosis by months or even years. There are two phases of GO: (1) An initial active inflammatory phase; and (2) A static or inactive phase. In the inactive phase, the long-lasting muscular edema along with the increased production of collagen leads ultimately to atrophy, fibrosis, and sclerosis of the extra-ocular musculature and subsequently to restrictive strabismus. GO rarely becomes active again, once it has become quiescent.

6. What are the clinical features of GO?

Graves' ophthalmopathy is usually bilateral with asymmetrical presentation in about 10–15% of cases. The unilateral presentation is rare in which case other causes need to be ruled out.

The most common symptoms and signs include:
- Ocular surface discomfort (ocular dryness and grittiness, photophobia, excessive tearing, and blurred vision)
- Changes in the appearance of the eye secondary to periorbital soft-tissue inflammation and congestion (sensation of retro-ocular pressure, conjunctival redness, and eyelid swelling)
- Aching with eye movement, restricted ocular motility, and double vision secondary to involvement of extraocular muscles
- Dysthyroid optic neuropathy caused by enlarged extraocular muscles at the orbital apex compressing the optic nerve.

7. What are the differential diagnoses of GO?

Alternative diagnosis should be considered when the presentation is unilateral or if the ocular signs are inconclusive in the absence of objective evidence of thyroid dysfunction. The other conditions which can affect the orbit could be inflammatory, neoplastic, infectious, vascular, or neuromuscular.
- Orbital pseudotumor or nonspecific orbital inflammation (~40%)
- Neoplasms include lymphomas, hamartomas, primary granulosa cell tumors, rhabdomyomas, liposarcomas, metastasis from breast, gastrointestinal, lung carcinomas, and melanomas (~20–40%)
- Other causes include infections, neuromuscular dysfunction, and vascular malformations (~10–15%)
- Specific orbital inflammation in the setting of sarcoidosis, systemic lupus erythematous, Crohn's disease, and scleroderma

8. What is the diagnosis of GO?

The diagnosis is based on clinical features:
- The presence of eye signs and symptoms
- The presence of thyroid autoimmunity
- The exclusion of an alternative diagnosis

9. What is the role of imaging in the diagnosis of GO?

Imaging is not routinely needed. It is valuable in case of diagnostic uncertainty such as unilateral presentation to identify patients at high risk of optic neuropathy and before planning for surgical decompression or orbital radiation. Among various imaging modalities available, CT of the orbits is widely used. The characteristic involvement of orbital muscles, where only muscle belly is involved sparing the ligaments, distinguishes GO from orbital pseudotumor where both are involved.

10. How do you approach this patient with GO?

- Assess quality of life (QoL) by GO-QoL questionnaire
- Assess disease activity by Clinical Activity Score (CAS)
- Assess disease severity by the European Group on Graves' Orbitopathy (EUGOGO) classification into mild, moderate-to-severe, and sight-threatening.

Each of these indices affect the aggressiveness of treatment.

11. What is GO-QoL questionnaire?

Graves' ophthalmopathy-quality of life is a well-validated tool, which assesses the effects of the disease and its treatment on QoL and psychosocial well-being. It consists of two subscales of GO-QoL: (1) Visual functioning; and (2) Appearance. Each subscale contains eight items and each item is scored on a three-point scale: 1—severely, 2—a little, and 3—not at all. It may serve as the primary outcome measure in clinical trials.

12. What is CAS?

It is a score that assesses the extent of acute inflammatory changes that imply disease activity in the eye (**Table 1**). It assesses soft-tissue changes in the eyelids, conjunctiva, and caruncle/plica. A CAS score of >3/7 is considered as active disease. On follow-up within 3 months, progression of GO can be assessed by changes in proptosis, ocular motility, and visual acuity (**Table 1**).

13. How do you assess disease severity?

The severity of the disease is assessed according to the EUGOGO classification (**Table 2**).

14. What is the diagnosis in this patient?

- Activity—inactive GO as CAS < 3
- Severity—mild, as the disease causes mild impairment in daily life, proptosis of <3 mm above the normal limit, and lid retraction of <2 mm with no diplopia

  This patient has a mild inactive GO with biochemically severe hyperthyroidism.

15. What are the risk factors for progression of GO in this case?

Biochemically severe hyperthyroidism.

16. What are the treatment options available for the management of GO?

- General measures
- *Immunosuppressive agents*: Intravenous or oral glucocorticoids and cyclosporine
- Orbital irradiation
- *Surgical options*: Orbital decompression, strabismus surgery, and eyelid surgery.

TABLE 1: Clinical activity score.

Inflammatory signs	Score
Pain	
Spontaneous retrobulbar pain	1
Gaze-evoked pain	1
Redness	
Redness of the conjunctiva	1
Redness of the eyelids	1
Swelling	
Swelling of the eyelids	1
Swelling of caruncle or plica	1
Chemosis	1
Maximum score assessed at that moment	7
On follow-up within 3 months, assess progression of GO by the following three parameters: 1. Increase in proptosis ≥2 mm 2. Decrease of ≥8° reduction in eye muscle motility in any direction 3. Decrease in visual acuity of more than one line on the Snellen chart (using pinhole)	1 1
Maximum score assessed over time	10

TABLE 2: Grading of severity of GO according to the EUGOGO classification.

Severity	Features
Mild GO	• Minor impact on quality of life insufficient to justify immunosuppressive or surgical treatment • They have one or more of the following: Minor lid retraction (<2 mm), mild soft-tissue involvement, proptosis <3 mm above normal for race and gender, no or intermittent diplopia, and corneal exposure responsive to lubricants
Moderate-to-severe GO	• Significant impact on quality of life, not threatening vision, requires immunosuppression, if active or surgical treatment if inactive • They have two or more of the following: Lid retraction ≥2 mm, moderate or severe soft-tissue involvement, proptosis ≥3 mm above normal for age and gender, and inconstant or constant diplopia
Sight-threatening GO	Patients with dysthyroid optic neuropathy and/or corneal breakdown

(GO: Graves' ophthalmopathy; EUGOGO: European Group on Graves' Orbitopathy)

17. What are the general measures for the management of GO and when is it indicated?

Graves' ophthalmopathy, whether overt or mild, develops ocular surface inflammatory disease and dry eye, while reduced tear production is seen only in active disease. Increased palpebral fissure width, lid lag, lagophthalmos, and exophthalmos cause drying of ocular surface. There is an increase in tear film osmolarity because of ocular surface evaporation, which is proportional to the degree of widening of palpable fissures. Reduced tear production is secondary to the presence of TSHR antibody on lacrimal glands leading to its dysfunction. Nonpreserved artificial tears and osmoprotective agents serve the purpose.

18. How do you manage this patient with mild inactive GO?

Prompt restoration of euthyroid status, with a close watch on preventing hypothyroidism, which may progress her GO.

Local or general measures—nonpreserved artificial tears and sunglasses help in photophobia and sleeping in semi-recumbent position improves tissue congestion in the morning.

No role for steroids as the disease is inactive causing mild impairment of QoL.

19. How do you manage thyroid disease in patients with GO?

Prompt restoration of euthyroidism is associated with improvement in GO, while uncontrolled hypothyroidism and late correction of hypothyroidism after radioactive iodine (RAI) treatment lead to occurrence of GO.

Antithyroid drugs and thyroidectomy do not change the natural history of GO. However, restoration of euthyroidism might have an indirect effect.

Radioactive iodine treatment is associated with an occurrence and progression of GO in at-risk individuals (smokers, preexisting GO, and recent-onset GO).

Antithyroid drug is the treatment of choice in this patient, as her chances of remission are highly likely and there are no contraindications to therapy. Patient should be monitored closely to avoid any hypothyroidism.

20. What is the role of selenium supplementation in mild GO?

Evidence suggests that increased generation of reactive oxygen species has a pathogenic role in GO. Selenocysteine has a major role in the cellular redox system. Role of selenium supplementation in the course of mild GO has been evaluated in a double-blind randomized controlled trial for a period of 6 months. The primary outcomes were changes in QoL assessment and ocular appearance. There was a significant change in the primary outcomes compared to placebo (ocular involvement 61% vs. 36% in the placebo group; $p < 0.001$). The improvement was maintained at 12 months after selenium withdrawal and the rate of progression to severe forms was significantly lower in selenium group (7% vs. 26% in the placebo group). No drug-related adverse events were reported. In long-standing inactive mild GO, selenium supplementation was not effective. The EUGOGO recommends selenium supplementation for 6 months in patients with recent-onset mild GO.

21. Is there a role of intravenous glucocorticoid therapy in this patient with mild inactive GO?

No. Intravenous methylprednisolone (IVMP) is indicated in mild inactive GO only, if there is significant impairment in QoL.

22. Is there a role for steroids if this patient develops intolerance to antithyroid drugs and is undergoing radioiodine ablation?

Oral corticosteroids are generally not indicated in patients with mild inactive GO undergoing RAI ablation.

23. Is there a role for steroids, if this patient has active mild GO and undergoing radioiodine ablation?

Yes. If the disease is active and the patient is undergoing RAI ablation, oral prednisone prophylaxis at a dose of 0.3–0.5 mg/kg body weight for a duration of 3 months is indicated to prevent the progression of GO.

24. What precautions need to be taken to avoid progression of GO after RAI?

Post-RAI hypothyroidism should be promptly recognized and treated as both hypothyroidism and hyperthyroidism increase the risk of progression of GO.

CASE 2

A 29-year-old male presents with thyrotoxic symptoms for a duration of 1 month. He complains of protrusion of the eyes right more than left, associated with redness, swelling of the eyelids, and spontaneous- and gaze-evoked retrobulbar pain and diplopia on looking toward right, there is no history of blurring of vision or color difference between eyes during the same time. He smokes about a pack of cigarette per day for the past 6–7 years. No family history of GD is present. His disease has a severe impairment in his QoL. He has no comorbidities.

On examination, he is alert, anxious with warm, moist extremities, and fine tremors. His vitals were PR: 110 beats/min, regular BP: 130/50 mm Hg, and RR: 16 breaths/min.

On ocular examination, erythema of the eyelids and conjunctiva, chemosis, swollen caruncle, and swollen eyelids are noted. All signs are more severe in right eye. Lid retraction is about 4 mm and proptosis is about 20 mm in left eye and 25 mm in right eye. Abduction is impaired in right eye. Visual acuity, color vision, and visual fields are normal.

His thyroid profile and technetium scan are suggestive of GD.

1. **What are the approach and diagnosis?**
   - Graves' ophthalmopathy-quality of life—impaired
   - Activity—CAS—7/7
   - Severity—moderate-to-severe (lid retraction >2 mm and proptosis >3 mm above normal and inconstant diplopia)
   - This patient should be referred to ophthalmology and endocrinology teams. Only mild cases of GO can be managed by a primary care physician

   This patient has moderate-to-severe active GO.

2. **What is the role of imaging in this case?**

   There is no role for imaging, as this patient has bilateral GO concomitant with thyroid dysfunction, which is diagnostic of GO. Imaging is indicated in case of unilateral or bilateral presentation with euthyroid status.

3. **What are the risk factors for progression of GO in this case?**

   Risk factors are male sex, smoking status, and biochemically severe hyperthyroidism.

4. **How do you manage thyroid status of this patient?**

   Prompt restoration of euthyroid status with antithyroid drugs. RAI treatment is contraindicated in moderate-to-severe active GO.

5. **How do you manage GO in this case?**
   - Counsel for smoking cessation
   - Intravenous methylprednisolone—intermediate-dose regimen
   - Assess for any contraindications for steroid therapy before initiating treatment

6. **What is the intravenous regimen for GO?**
   - *Intermediate-dose regimen*: Up to 0.5 g of methylprednisolone once weekly for 6 weeks followed by 0.25 g once weekly for 6 weeks (4.5 g cumulative dose)—recommended for most cases of moderate-to-severe GO.
   - *High-dose regimen*: Up to 0.75 g of methylprednisolone once weekly for 6 weeks followed by 0.5 g once weekly for 6 weeks (cumulative dose of 7.5 g)—recommended for the worst cases within the spectrum of moderate-to-severe GO.

     Cumulative doses should not exceed 8 g. Doses >8 g have been associated with hepatotoxicity and cardiovascular morbidity and mortality.

7. **What are the contraindications for intravenous glucocorticoid therapy?**

   Contraindications are uncontrolled diabetes mellitus and hypertension, recent viral hepatitis, significant hepatic dysfunction, severe cardiovascular morbidity, glaucoma, and psychiatric disorders.

Assessment of liver enzymes, viral markers of hepatitis, hepatic ultrasound, and glycemic status should be assessed before initiating therapy.

Liver enzymes, blood glucose, and blood pressure should be monitored monthly after initiating treatment.

8. How do you monitor these patients on IVMP?
- Assess for improvement in CAS. A reduction of more than two points is considered favorable treatment response in clinical trials.
- Assess for adverse effects of IVMP. Monitor liver enzymes, blood pressure, and blood glucose every month.

9. How do you manage this patient, if he is not responding to steroids or has a relapse after initial therapy?
Several second-line options are available:
- Second course of IVMP—contraindicated, if patients were intolerant to steroids during the first course
- Orbital radiation therapy, as monotherapy or along with oral steroid cover, if no adverse effects
- Cyclosporine (5–7.5 mg/kg body weight for 12 months) + oral glucocorticoids (starting dose of 100–60 mg prednisone with tapering over 3 months)
- Rituximab (1 g twice at 2-week interval)

10. What are the indications for orbital radiation therapy?
Orbital radiation has a suppressive effect on activated intraorbital lymphocytes and fibroblasts leading to a decrease in the production of cytokines and glycosaminoglycans. It can be given as a monotherapy or as a combination therapy with glucocorticoids.

Monotherapy: If glucocorticoids are contraindicated in active GO of recent onset, specifically, if the patient has diplopia as a problem.

Combination therapy with oral glucocorticoids: As a second-line treatment, if there is a recurrence following intravenous glucocorticoids and if the patient is not willing for a second course of IV glucocorticoids or if there were side effects associated with their use. Combination therapy is more effective than either treatment alone.

Protocol: 20 Gy delivered in 10 fractions over 2 weeks along with a short course of glucocorticoids to avoid transient exacerbation.

It is not recommended for patients younger than 35 years of age, as safety data is not available in this age group.

Rare side effects include radiation-induced cataracts and radiation-induced retinopathy. It is better avoided in patients with diabetes.

11. What are the newer treatment options for GO?

Teprotumumab, a monoclonal insulin-like growth factor 1 receptor (IGF-1R) antibody, has been shown to have significantly reduced the proptosis (>2 mm) compared to placebo. It is the first drug approved by the Food and Drug Administration (FDA) for the treatment of GO.

12. Few months later, his GO became inactive, but is worried about his appearance, diplopia, and corneal exposure because of inadequate closure of eyelids in the night. What do you advise him now?

He is now a candidate for rehabilitative surgery. Orbital decompression improves proptosis, correction of strabismus surgery improves ocular alignment and restores binocular vision, and lid lengthening decreases corneal exposure.

13. What is the role of surgical management in GO?

Surgery has a role in rehabilitation to improve the QoL in patients with inactive GO and as emergency decompression of the orbit in dysthyroid optic neuropathy.

Three surgical modalities are available: (1) Orbital decompression, (2) Correction of strabismus, and (3) Eyelid adjustment surgery. They are performed in this order, if the patient requires more than one surgery.

14. What is orbital decompression surgery and what are the indications and complications?

Orbital decompression consists of expansion of the bony boundaries of the orbits (medial, inferomedial, lateral, and deep lateral) or orbital fat removal or both. This approach reduces the raised intraorbital pressure and reduces the proptosis.

Indications: Rehabilitation in inactive GO, in patients with dysthyroid optic neuropathy, either urgently or after a course of IV glucocorticoids for 2 weeks and globe subluxation.

Complications: New or worsened motility problems, which develop in 0–60% of patients. Other complications include blindness, orbital cellulitis, cerebrospinal fluid (CSF) leak, cerebral hepatoma, cutaneous sensory loss, nasolacrimal outflow obstruction, and eyelid malposition.

CASE 3

A 42-year-old male, nonsmoker, underwent radioiodine ablation for Graves' hyperthyroidism 6 months ago and has lost to follow-up. He now presents with history of pain in the right eye and swelling and redness in and around the eye along with blurring of vision. He had no eye symptoms at the time of RAI. He also gained significant weight during this period.

On examination, patient is lethargic and skin is cold and dry. His vitals are PR: 60 beats/min and BP: 130/90 mm Hg.

Right eye examination: Erythema of the conjunctiva and eyelids, chemosis, swollen eyelids, and swollen caruncle are noted. He has restriction of extraocular movements and diminished visual acuity in the right eye. Fundus examination is normal.

His serum TSH: 124 µIU/mL, T4: 3.5 µg/dL and T3: 74 ng/dL.

1. What is the diagnosis of this patient?

This patient has a severe sight-threatening GO.

2. What are the risk factors for GO in this patient?

Overt hypothyroidism is the risk factor for developing GO in this patient. Monitoring and prompt treatment of hypothyroidism after RAI ablation is essential to prevent development of GO.

3. Is there a role of imaging in this patient?

Yes. As this patient has sight-threatening GO, orbital imaging would help in better planning for the surgery by visualizing the disturbed anatomy and the extent of the disease.

4. How do you manage severe sight-threatening GO?

Sight-threatening GO is an endocrine emergency. IVMP for 2 weeks followed by prompt decompression is the treatment approach.

High-dose IVMP 500–1,000 mg for 3 consecutive days or on alternate day during the first 2 weeks results in improvement of vision in 40% of patients.

If the response is poor or absent, then urgent orbital decompression surgery is recommended after 2 weeks.

CONCLUSION

Graves' orbitopathy occurs in patients with Graves' disease and is an autoimmune disease of retro-ocular tissue. Complications can be serious and sight-threatening. It can precede the onset of thyrotoxicosis. The treatment is steroids and surgical decompression. Newer therapies like teprotumumab have been approved by FDA.

SUGGESTED READINGS

1. Barrio-Barrio J, Sabater AL, Bonet-Farriol E, Velázquez-Villoria Á, Galofré JC. Graves' Ophthalmopathy: VISA versus EUGOGO Classification, Assessment, and Management. J Ophthalmol. 2015;2015:24912.
2. Bartalena L, Baldeschi L, Boboridis K, Eckstein A, Kahaly GJ, Marcocci C, et al. The 2016 European Thyroid Association/European Group on Graves' Orbitopathy Guidelines for the Management of Graves' Orbitopathy. Eur Thyroid J. 2016;5:9-26.

3. Boddu N, Jumani M, Wadhwa V, Bajaj G, Faas F. Not All Orbitopathy Is Graves': Discussion of Cases and Review of Literature. Front Endocrinol (Lausanne). 2017;8:184.

4. Douglas RS. Teprotumumab, an insulin-like growth factor-1 receptor antagonist antibody, in the treatment of active thyroid eye disease: a focus on proptosis. Eye (Lond). 2019;33: 183-90.

5. Hiromatsu Y, Eguchi H, Tani J, Kasaoka M, Teshima Y. Graves' ophthalmopathy: epidemiology and natural history. Intern Med. 2014;53:353-60.

6. Marcocci C, Bartalena L, Bogazzi F, Bruno-Bossio G, Lepri A, Pinchera A. Orbital radiotherapy combined with high dose systemic glucocorticoids for Graves' ophthalmopathy is more effective than radiotherapy alone: results of a prospective randomized study. J Endocrinol Invest. 1991;14:853-60.

7. Marcocci C, Kahaly GJ, Krassas GE, Bartalena L, Prummel M, Stahl M, et al. Selenium and the course of mild Graves' orbitopathy. N Engl J Med. 2011;364:1920-31.

8. Marcocci C, Watt T, Altea MA, Rasmussen AK, Feldt-Rasmussen U, Orgiazzi J, et al. Fatal and non-fatal adverse events of glucocorticoid therapy for Graves' orbitopathy: a questionnaire survey among members of the European Thyroid Association. Eur J Endocrinol. 2012;166: 247-53.

9. Perros P, Dickinson J. Ophthalmopathy. In: Braveman LE, David S (Eds). Werner and Ingbar's The Thyroid, 10th edition. Lippincott: Williams & Wilkins; 2013. pp. 369-70.

10. Ross DS, Burch HB, Cooper DS, Greenlee MC, Laurberg P, Maia AL, et al. 2016 American Thyroid Association Guidelines for Diagnosis and Management of Hyperthyroidism and Other Causes of Thyrotoxicosis. Thyroid. 2016;26:1343-421.

11. Wiersinga WM, Kahaly GJ. Graves' Orbitopathy: A Multidisciplinary Approach—Questions and Answers. Basel: Karger; 2017. pp. 33-40.

12. Wiersinga WM. Quality of life in Graves' ophthalmopathy. Best Pract Res Clin Endocrinol Metab. 2012;26:359-70.

11

CHAPTER   ## Osteogenesis Imperfecta

Anjana Hulse

INTRODUCTION

Osteogenesis imperfecta is a group of inherited disorders of connective tissues characterized by bone fragility of varying degrees. Most common defect is mutations resulting in qualitative and quantitative abnormalities of type I collagen. Children with osteogenesis imperfecta often present with frequent fractures, skeletal abnormalities, hearing defects, dental abnormalities, and short stature. Early diagnosis and pharmacological intervention helps to minimize morbidity among these children.

CASE HISTORY

A 1.2-year-old boy presented with history of uncontrollable crying. On examination, he was noted to have a swelling in his right lower limb. On further evaluation, it was noted that he had sustained a fracture of right tibia. There was no history of trauma or any kind of injury. He was the only child of a nonconsanguineous couple. Antenatal scan had revealed short femur but no other abnormality. He was born at term without any complications, weighing 2,900 g. He was thriving normally during the first few months of his life.

There was a past history of fracture of right tibia at the age of 9 months following a trivial injury and a fracture of left femur after a fall at 1 year. Both the times the fracture was treated conservatively. On further enquiry about the family it was noticed that his mother was short (142 cm) and had blue sclera (**Fig. 1**). She had sustained a fracture of right forearm a few years ago when she fell while getting down from a bus. The father was 175 cm tall and had no fractures in the past.

On detailed examination, the child was short for his age measuring 70 cm (<3rd centile). He weighed 7,500 g (<3rd centile). He had triangular face and blue sclera (**Fig. 2**). There was a swelling over the right lower limb (tibia). Rest of the examination was normal. A radiograph of the right lower limb revealed severe osteopenia and an undisplaced fracture of shaft of tibia. Further evaluation with the radiographs suggested generalized severe osteopenia. His DEXA scan revealed bone mineral density (BMD) of 0.615 (whole body)

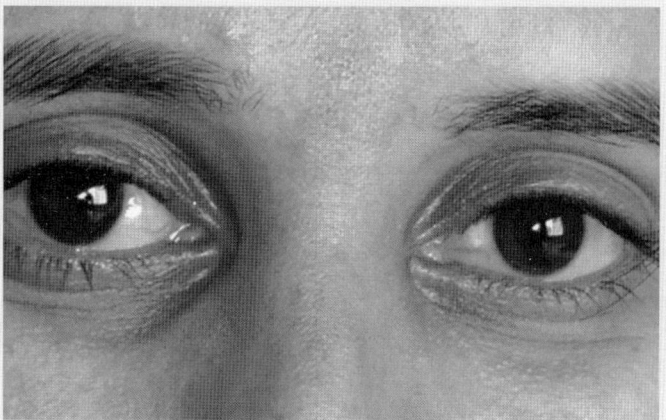

FIG. 1: Blue sclera in the mother. (*For color version, see plate 5*)

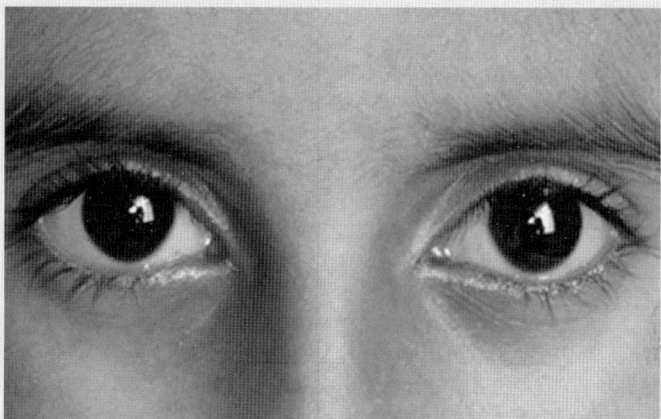

FIG. 2: Blue sclera. (*For color version, see plate 5*)

and 0.780 (spine) g/cm^2. Laboratory investigations including serum calcium, phosphorus, alkaline phosphatase, renal function, and fractional excretion of phosphorus was normal, but vitamin D was low (11 ng/mL).

Based on the above mentioned features such as frequent fractures, blue sclera, osteopenia on radiographs, and possible family history of mild variant of osteogenesis imperfecta (OI) in the mother, a clinical diagnosis of OI (type I) was made. The patient had a hearing screen done which was normal. He was treated conservatively for the fracture of right tibia. After the fracture healed, he was started on cyclical infusion of pamidronate. The first infusion was started when he was 1.4 years. He received pamidronate infusion 0.5 mg/kg/day (given over 4 h) for three consecutive days every 3 months during the first year of therapy. During the first year of therapy, there was a fragility fracture of mandible after an injury which was managed conservatively. He also developed gingivitis, gum bleeds, and tooth decay (**Fig. 3**). He was being treated with supportive therapy for the same by a pediatric dentist. During

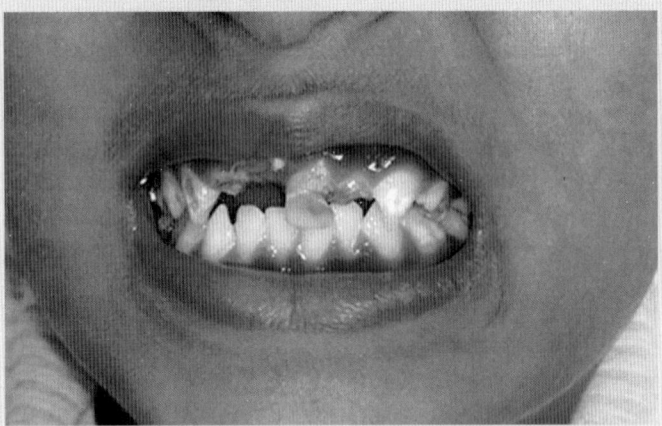

FIG. 3: Dentinogenesis imperfecta. (***For color version, see plate 5***)

the second year of therapy, he received pamidronate infusion 1 mg/kg/day for 3 consecutive days every 4 months. Thereafter, he received two more cycles of pamidronate infusion at an interval of 6 months. Currently, he is 4.5 years and has not had any fracture in the past 2 years. He had annual BMD assessed which showed gradual improvement over the last 2 years of bisphosphonate therapy. There was improvement in his growth. However, he still remains below two standard deviations (SD) on the growth chart.

DISCUSSION

Osteogenesis imperfecta (brittle bone disease) is a genetic disorder characterized by extreme bone fragility and osteoporosis which often predisposes the patients to frequent fractures. The disorder has been attributed to defect in type I collagen synthesis. Various forms of OI characterized by different genetic mutations and variable clinical features have been identified. The prevalence of OI is about 1:20,000 live births of which about 50% of the cases belong to milder varieties of OI. Diagnosis of mild OI can be challenging.

Clinical Features of Osteogenesis Imperfecta

The clinical features of OI may be variable. Wormian bones in the skull may be seen in about 60% of the cases. Generalized osteoporosis is a constant finding and this may be worsened by immobilization due to fractures or surgery and lack of physical activity. Mid shaft fractures are common but metaphyseal fractures which are pathognomonic of nonaccidental injury in children can also occur. Other clinical features that may be present are joint hyperlaxity, muscle weakness, chronic bone pain, and skull deformities (e.g., posterior flattening) due to bone fragility. Hearing is affected in some cases. Respiratory complications secondary to kyphoscoliosis are common. About 30% of the patients with OI may develop dentinogenesis imperfecta where there is abnormal dentin but enamel is normal. Basilar invagination is a potentially fatal condition associated with OI. In perinatally lethal form (type II), there may be findings of crumpled and deformed long bones and deficient ossification of skull and facial bones on antenatal scan. This type may be associated with neuronal migration defects and white matter changes. Perinatal mortality is common. Except in severe forms, life expectancy in OI is same as that of normal population.

Nonskeletal Complications in Osteogenesis Imperfecta

Hypoacusis may be present in about 50% of the cases of OI. Hypercalciuria may be present in some cases but it does not impair renal function. In individuals with severe OI with kyphoscoliosis, respiratory complications may be frequently encountered. Increased capillary fragility may cause frequent bruising in some patients. Constipation and hernia are also common in these patients. Joint hyperlaxity leading to dislocation and flat foot are other associated problems. Dental malocclusion and dentinogenesis imperfecta are common in some types of OI. One of the less common but a serious complication is basilar invagination.

Radiological Findings in Osteogenesis Imperfecta

Generalized hypomineralization is a consistent finding on the radiographs of patients with OI. Thin cortices and metaphyseal flaring may be seen. Children with OI often present with long bone fractures. Shaft fractures are commonly seen on radiographs. In some cases, metaphyseal fractures may also be seen. Fractures of different ages are seen in this condition. Wormian skull bones, platybasia, and triradiate pelvis are associated findings in some cases. Bone fragility in the spine may lead to fractures. They commonly present as deformed vertebrae with a biconcave shape due to the pressure exerted by the intervertebral disks at the endplate.

Diagnosis of Osteogenesis Imperfecta

Osteogenesis imperfecta is diagnosed based on the above mentioned clinical and radiological features. The diagnosis can be confirmed by genotyping of COL1A1 and/or COL1A2 and other genetic defects. Failure to detect a mutation does not rule out OI. Occasionally, biopsy of the iliac crest and histological examination of the bone may be necessary for diagnosis and subclassification of this disorder.

If a Fetus is Affected, What Findings may be Seen on Prenatal Ultrasonography?

Osteogenesis imperfecta is one of the most common skeletal dysplasia detected on antenatal scan. During the first trimester, OI may be diagnosed based on morphological features seen on scan and by chorionic villous sampling. During the second trimester, bowing and deformities of the long bones, short femur, and rib fractures may be seen. Decreased echoes from calvarium are also a common finding.

Classification of Osteogenesis Imperfecta

In 1979, Sillence proposed a classification of OI (OI types I to IV). OI type II was subsequently subdivided in OI type II-A, B, and C based on radiological features. Later, Glorieux and Rauch expanded this classification to OI types V to VIII based on unknown genetic defects and presumed autosomal recessive or dominant inheritance. The first genetic cause of OI that was detected was an internal deletion in a collagen gene *(COL1A1)*. *COL1A1/A2* accounts for majority of cases of OI. Newer classifications mainly based on genetic defects have led to confusion among the clinicians as these groups are not mutually exclusive. Therefore, in 2009, the International Nomenclature group for Constitutional Disorders ICHG of the Skeleton (INCDS) (published as 2010 Nosology), classified the known OI syndromes into five groups as illustrated in **Table 1**.

TABLE 1: Baseline laboratory examinations.

OI syndrome	Type	Clinical features	Gene	Inheritance
Nondeforming OI with blue sclerae	I	Most common type (1 in 25,000 live births), distinctly blue sclera, increased bone fragility, conductive hearing loss, dentinogenesis imperfecta	*CAL1A1, COL1A2*	A1
Common variable OI with normal sclerae	IV	Sclerae normal, increased bone fragility with variable severity, posterior fossa compression syndromes due to basilar impression is common	• *CAL1A1, COL1A2, WNT1* • *CRTAP, PPIB, SP7* • *PLS3*	• AD • AR • XL
OI with calcification in interosseous membranes	V	Progressive calcification of the interosseous membranes in the forearms and legs, moderate-to-severe bone fragility, bone histomorphometry shows coarse mesh-like lamellation	*IFITM5*	AD
Progressively deforming	III	Multiple fractures starting from newborn period, progressive deformity, popcorn appearance of metaphyses, chest wall deformities, Wormian bones	• *CAL1A1, COL1A2* • *BMP1, CRTAP, FKBP10, LEPRE1, PLOD2, PPIB, SERPINF1, SERPINH1, TMEM38B, WNT1, CREB3L1*	• AD • AR

Continued

Continued

OI syndrome	Type	Clinical features	Gene	Inheritance
Perinatally lethal OI	II	The most severe form. Antenatal scan may show crumpled and deformed long bones, deficient ossification of facial and skull bones, rib fractures, bead like ribs, some cases may have brain migration defects and/or white matter changes. Perinatal mortality is common. Rarely survive into adult life	• *CAL1A1, COL1A2* • *CRTAP, LEPRE1, PPIB*	• AD • AR

(OI: osteogenesis imperfecta)

Pathophysiology of Osteogenesis Imperfecta

In most cases of OI, heterozygous loss of function mutations has been identified in one of the two genes *(COL1A1, COL1A2)*. These genes code for procollagen subunits alpha-1 and alpha-2 which form collagen I in various tissues such as bones, sclerae, dentin, skin, ligaments, and tendons. Type I collagen is a triple helical structure which contains one alpha 2 and two alpha 1 polypeptide chains. Mutations (insertion, duplication, frame shift or point mutations) within *COL1A1* or *COL2A2* genes transmitted as an autosomal dominant trait, lead to reduction in the amount of collagen synthesized or alter its structure, leading to low bone mass and increased susceptibility for fracture. The severity of the clinical presentation depends upon the effect of mutation. Mutations in *COL1A1* or *COL1A2* that lead to decreased amounts of normal collagen cause the mild phenotype seen in type I OI. In contrast, the lethal phenotypes seen in type II OI are caused by mutations leading to disruption in triple helical structure of collagen type I. Other mutations that result in structural protein defects cause moderate (type IV) and severe forms of OI. More than 800 mutations have been identified within *COL1A1* and *COL1A2*.

Syndromes Resembling Osteogenesis Imperfecta

The following are the syndromes resembling OI:
- Congenital brittle bones with rhizomelia
- Congenital brittle bones with redundant callus
- Osteoporosis-pseudoglioma syndrome
- Congenital brittle bones with microcephaly and cataracts
- Congenital brittle bones with optic atrophy, retinopathy, and severe psychomotor retardation
- Congenital brittle bones with craniosynostosis and ocular proptosis
- Congenital brittle bones with congenital joint contractures
- Congenital brittle bones with mineralization defect

Pharmacological Treatment Options for Osteogenesis Imperfecta

The medical treatment of patients with OI is aimed at prevention of frequent fractures and the morbidity associated with it and improvement of linear growth. Treatment of fractures by using appropriate orthopedic measures is very important too. Appropriate physical therapy to improve bone and muscle strength should be encouraged.

For children with OI, biochemical status of calcium and vitamin D should be assessed. Supplementation with calcium and vitamin D preparations should be provided to optimize the levels. Pharmacological therapy using bisphosphonates is now used all over the world for moderate-to-severe OI and it has become an important part of management of OI. Even though growth hormone (GH) has been used in some research settings in selected patients, routine use of GH for OI patients is not recommended. Other drugs which are being tried in OI include teriparatide and denosumab.

Bisphosphonate Therapy in Osteogenesis Imperfecta

Historically, pamidronate is the bisphosphonate which is commonly used in treatment of OI. Children with OI with frequent fractures (>2/year) and deformities of long bones or vertebrae are the candidates for treatment irrespective of their BMD status or genetic and clinical type of their OI. Standard treatment recommendation includes pamidronate 0.5 mg/kg/day as intravenous infusion for 3 consecutive days every 2 months for children <2 years, 0.75 mg/kg/day for 3 days every 3 months for children between 2 to 3 years and 1 mg/kg/day (maximum 60 mg/day) for 3 days every 4 months for children over 3 years. It has been safely used even in infants in severe cases. Modified versions of this protocol are used in some centers. Duration of treatment with bisphosphonates may vary depending on the response to therapy. Because of the persistence of bisphosphonates in the bone and their long-term effects, it is suggested that the therapy is continued for 2–4 years. Thereafter, regular follow-up with BMD is necessary to assess the need for further therapy with bisphosphonate.

Bisphosphonates increase the vertebral bone mass and size; thereby, reducing vertebral compression. In the iliac crest, the medication increases the cortical thickness and trabecular number. In metacarpals, cortical thickness is enhanced. Bisphosphonate therapy in children with OI is known to increase lumbar spine BMD, decrease fracture rate, and improve vertebral compression fractures. There will be significant improvement in bone pain when treatment with bisphosphonates is started. Height z scores will increase in children when treatment is started before 3 years of age.

Bisphosphonates may cause transient hypocalcemia, flu-like reaction of fever, rash, headache, and vomiting, especially during the first cycle. This can be treated with paracetamol. Serum calcium, phosphorus, alkaline phosphatase, and renal function should be checked before starting

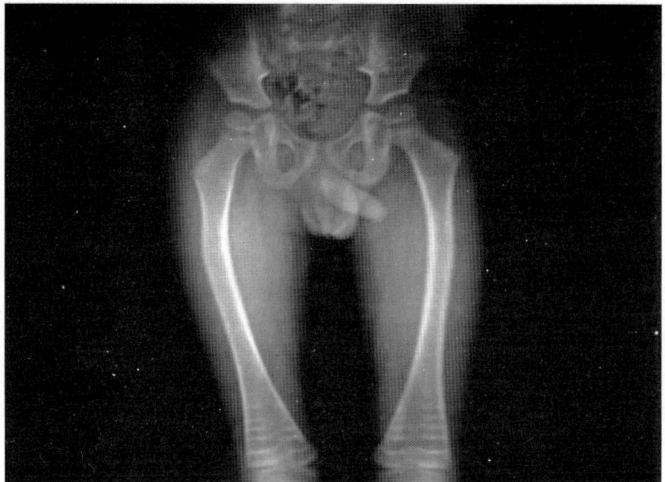

FIG. 4: Metaphyseal bands in a child on cyclical pamidronate infusion.

bisphosphonate infusion. Vitamin D and calcium levels should be optimized in children with OI. Osteonecrosis of the jaw has been reported in some cases.

Other bisphosphonates such as zoledronic acid are used in some centers. Oral alendronate at a dose of 1 mg/kg/day is reported to be as effective as intravenous pamidronate, although data are limited on gastrointestinal tolerability and absorption of the drug in children.

Figure 4 is a Radiograph of this Patient. What do the Horizontal Lines in Figure 2 Indicate?

The horizontal lines or zebra lines seen in the radiograph are "metaphyseal bands." Differential remodeling of the bone due to cyclic antiosteoclastic activity of the bisphosphonates leads to these lines. These lines correspond to increased and normal bone mineralization during bisphosphonate treatment.

Growth Hormone in Osteogenesis Imperfecta

The use of GH in children with OI is controversial. It is never used as first-line therapy in OI. In terms of linear growth, some may be "responders" and some "nonresponders." Careful selection of the patients is needed to get the maximum benefit. There is limited literature on use of GH in children with OI. The existing literature supports use of GH in selected patients with moderate forms of OI with quantitative collagen defects to increase their linear growth, improve BMD, and reduce fracture risk. It should be kept in mind that in pre-existing scoliosis or bone deformities, use of GH may worsen the condition. OI is not a licensed condition for the use of GH and this has to be explained to the patients before starting therapy. GH does not seem to be useful in children with severe form of OI.

Newer Treatment Modalities for Osteogenesis Imperfecta

Antiresorptive agents, anabolic drugs, gene therapy, stem cell therapy, and bone marrow transplantation are being tried in research settings for treating patients with OI.

Differentiation of Osteogenesis Imperfecta from Nonaccidental Injury

Elaborate history including family history and thorough examination is important in distinguishing OI from nonaccidental injury. Radiologically, there may be some overlap between the two conditions as no type of fracture excludes OI. Certain features are thought to be highly specific in nonaccidental injury. These include fractures of the metaphyses, ribs, scapulae, vertebrae, the outer ends of the clavicles, bilateral fractures, fractures of different ages, complex fractures of the skull, and injuries of the fingers in nonwalking children. Absence of external injury such as bruises, history consistent with fracture site but the force too minimal to cause fracture or fractures sustained in different environments may point toward OI rather than nonaccidental injury. Though wormian bones and generalized osteopenia are common in OI and can help distinguish the two entities, in infants with OI, fractures may be present in a normal skeleton (without osteoporosis) which may, sometime, pose diagnostic dilemma for clinicians. In these scenarios where clinical and radiological findings are inconclusive, fibroblast culture from skin biopsy can be used to distinguish the two conditions.

Do Patients with Osteogenesis Imperfecta have a Tendency to Malignant Hyperthermia under Anesthesia?

It is a myth. Some patients with OI may have hypermetabolic state, with excessive diaphoresis, increased oxygen consumption, and elevated thyroxine levels. They may develop hyperthermia but malignant hyperthermia is rare.

CONCLUSION

Osteogenesis imperfecta is one of the commonest inheritable disorders which presents with varying severity. Prognosis is variable depending on the severity of the illness. Early diagnosis and treatment helps in minimizing fractures and morbidity.

SUGGESTED READINGS

1. Lifshitz F. Pediatric Endocrinology. 1st ed. Hoboken: Taylor and Francis; 2013.
2. Marini JC, Bordenick S, Heavner G, et al. The growth hormone and somatomedin axis in short children with osteogenesis imperfecta. J Clin Endocrinol Metab. 1993;76:251-56.
3. Monti E, Mottes M, Fraschini P, et al. Current and emerging treatments for the management of osteogenesis imperfecta. Therapeutics and Clinical Risk Management. 2010;6:367-81.
4. Rauch F, Glorieux FH. Osteogenesis imperfecta. Lancet 2004;363:1377-85.
5. Sillence D, Briody J, Ault J, et al. Factors which influence the efficacy of growth hormone in 15 children with osteogenesis imperfecta types I and IV. Sixth International Conference on Osteogenesis Imperfecta; 1996 Sep 19–21; Utrecht, The Netherlands; 1996.

12

CHAPTER **Renal Tubular Acidosis**

Chirag Umesh, Pramila Kalra

CASE 1

A 37-year-old female presented with fracture neck of the right femur following trivial trauma. She had history of diffuse body aches and proximal muscle weakness for the last 6 months. There was no history of recurrent pain in abdomen, diarrhea, steatorrhea, polyuria, or periodic paralysis. She had history of poor exposure to sunlight and deficient intake of dairy products. There was no past history of fracture, renal stone disease, gallstone disease, or pancreatitis. She had no history of use of glucocorticoids in any form, alternative medications, bisphosphonates, or calcium and vitamin D preparations. However, she complained of difficulty in swallowing and foreign body sensations in her eyes. She had two live children and the last child birth was 3 years earlier and she continues to menstruate regularly. Family history was noncontributory. Her blood pressure was 100/60 mm Hg. She had genu varum, kyphoscoliosis, diffuse bony tenderness, proximal muscle weakness, and severe attrition of her teeth with pigmentation. Her eyes were suffused and tongue was dry. Movements at left hip joint were restricted and painful.

On investigations, hemoglobin was 10.2 g/dL, serum creatinine was 1.2 mg/dL [estimated glomerular filtration rate (eGFR) was 40 mL/min/1.73 m^2], Na$^+$ was 145 mEq/L, K$^+$ was 2.8 mEq/L, corrected calcium was 9 mg/dL, phosphorus was 3.0 mg/dL, alkaline phosphatase was 919 IU/L (normal <128 IU/L), intact parathyroid hormone (iPTH) was 220 pg/mL (normal: 15–65 pg/mL), and 25-hydroxyvitamin D [25(OH)D] was 30 ng/mL (normal: 30–70 ng/mL). Arterial blood gas analysis revealed pH 7.28, calculated anion gap was 11 mEq/L, and corresponding urine pH was 6.5. Antinuclear antibody was present (speckled pattern, 4+). Her urine biochemistry revealed specific gravity 1.004, urine osmolality 175 mOsm/L, and pH 7.0.

Schirmer's test was positive and lip biopsy was consistent with Sjögren's syndrome. On further evaluation, the patient had a high urine anion gap (UAG) of +23. Repeated urine studies showed persistent alkaline urine (pH range: 6.5–7) with no evidence of glycosuria or phosphaturia. These findings were consistent with distal renal tubular acidosis (dRTA).

With this profile a diagnosis of distal renal tubular acidosis secondary to Sjögrens syndrome was diagnosed. The patient was initiated on sodium bicarbonate, potassium citrate, and calcium carbonate tablets. With this treatment, her bone pain resolved, proximal myopathy improved, and she was able to walk with support.

CASE 2

A 2-year-old child, who was born out of full-term pregnancy and uncompli-cated delivery, was admitted for fever, vomiting, and severe dehydration. She was noted to have short stature and genu varum. Radiographic studies revealed rachitic rosary and other changes compatible with rickets. Laboratory evaluation revealed, hypophosphatemia (0.51 mmol/L), increased alkaline phosphatase (600 U/L), hyperchloremic metabolic acidosis (Cl 114 mEq/L with HCO_3 6.9 mEq/L), generalized aminoaciduria, glucosuria, hyperphosphaturia (246.4 mEq/24 h/m²), hypercalciuria (42.5 mEq/24 h/m²), low-molecular-weight proteinuria (0.85 g/24 h/m²), serum ceruloplasmin, gamma-globulin, tyrosine, and ammonia. Family history indicated several other family members had bowed legs and rickets. Subsequently, other members of the family were studied in an attempt to make a specific diagnosis. The child was treated with $1,25(OH)_2$ vitamin D, sodium phosphate and potassium citrate. The rachitic changes improved during the following year. The patient continued to have reduced growth.

Similar findings were seen in three members and a diagnosis of familial Fanconi syndrome leading to proximal renal tubular acidosis was made.

What is Renal Tubular Acidosis?

Renal tubular acidosis may be defined as a group of disorders characterized primarily by the impairment of the ability of the kidney to handle principally hydrogen, bicarbonate ions, and other glomerular filtrate products of the body, which can occur due to multiple etiologies and can lead to a heterogeneous spectrum of clinical laboratory manifestations.

What are the Types of Renal Tubular Acidosis (RTA)?

- Type 1—distal tubular defect
- Type 2—proximal tubular defect
- Type 3—mixed defects
- Type 4—hyporeninemic hypoaldosteronism

How do you Broadly Classify the Etiology of RTA?

The etiology of RTA can be broadly classified into inherited and acquired causes.

The inherited causes may include defects of renal transporter proteins or may be a part of metabolic disorders.

The acquired causes may include drugs, systemic diseases, heavy metal poisoning, and renal transplantation.

What is the Common Characteristic Feature of RTA?

Renal tubular acidosis is characterized by normal anion gap metabolic acidosis and generally diagnosed in the presence of normal renal function.

What are the Other Causes of Normal Anion Gap Acidosis?

The other causes of normal anion gap acidosis are described in **Table 1**.

What are the Other Disorders Causing Similar Presentation in Children (as in Case 2)?

- Primary hyperparathyroidism (PHPT)
- Severe osteomalacia with secondary hyperparathyroidism
- Hypophosphatemic osteomalacia
- Osteogenesis imperfecta

What is Type 1 RTA? What are the Clinical and Laboratory Manifestations of this Type 1 RTA?

Type 1 RTA is caused by defective functioning of the distal renal tubule primarily leading to impairment of renal handling of H^+ ions and other glomerular filtrate products leading to normal anion gap acidosis.

The clinical manifestations may be due to bone disease such as stunted growth in children fragility fractures and nephrolithiasis. It may be due to secondary metabolic abnormalities associated with hypokalemia such as muscle aches, quadriparesis, and arrhythmias. It may also be asymptomatic.

TABLE 1: Causes of normal anion gap acidosis.

Gastrointestinal bicarbonate loss	• Diarrhea • Small bowel drainage • Drugs—calcium chloride, magnesium sulfate, and cholestyramine
Drug-induced hyperkalemia (with renal insufficiency)	• Potassium-sparing diuretics—amiloride, triamterene, spironolactone, ACE inhibitors, ARB, NSAID, heparin, and trimethoprim
Others	• Acid loads (hyperalimentation and ammonium chloride) • Expansion acidosis (rapid saline administration)

(ACE: angiotensin-converting enzyme; ARB: angiotensin receptor blocker; NSAID: nonsteroidal anti-inflammatory drug)

The typical metabolic abnormalities may be hypokalemia, hypercalciuria, hypocitraturia, low ammonia excretion, and inappropriately high urine pH > 5.5.

What are the Major Causes of Distal RTA?

The major causes of distal RTA are given in **Table 2**.

What is Type 2 RTA? What are the Clinical and Laboratory Manifestations of this Type 2 RTA?

Type 2 RTA is caused by defective functioning of the proximal renal tubule primarily leading to impairment of renal handling of H^+ ions and other glomerular filtrate products leading to normal anion gap acidosis.

The clinical manifestations may be related to electrolyte imbalance such as vomiting and dehydration. It may also lead to malnutrition and stunted growth related to loss of amino acids and glucose.

The laboratory manifestations may include glucosuria, aminoaciduria, and phosphaturia.

What are the Causes of Type 2 RTA?

The causes of type RTA are illustrated in **Table 3**.

What is Mixed (Type 3) RTA? What are the Clinical Findings in Children?

Type 3 RTA, also referred to as mixed RTA, is a rare autosomal recessive disorder that has features of both distal and proximal RTA. It is due to an inherited carbonic anhydrase (CA) 2 deficiency.

Because CA2 is widely expressed, mutations of the *CA2* gene result in a syndrome with multiple clinical findings including mixed RTA, osteopetrosis, cerebral calcification, and mental retardation.

TABLE 2: Major causes of distal RTA.

Inherited	Salient features
• SLC4A1 mutation	• Autosomal dominant
• ATP6VB1	• Autosomal recessive—early hearing loss
• ATP6V0A4	• Autosomal recessive
• WDR72	• Dental abnormalities
• Ehlers–Danlos syndrome	
Acquired	
• Drugs—amphotericin B and lithium	• More common in adults
• Autoimmune disorders—SLE and Sjögren's syndrome	• Rare in children
• Obstructive uropathy	• Impaired distal tubular protein function and mineralocorticoid function

(RTA: renal tubular acidosis; SLE: systemic lupus erythematosus)

TABLE 3: Causes of type 2 renal tubular acidosis (RTA).

Inherited	Salient features
• SLCA4—NBCe1 protein mutation • Autosomal dominant form—unidentified mutation • Dent disease • Lowe syndrome • Cystinosis • Tyrosinemia type 1	• Cataract, glaucoma, and familial migraine • Metabolic acidosis and short stature • Bony deformities • Oculocerebrorenal syndrome
Acquired • Drugs—aminoglycosides, cisplatin, ifosfamide, valproic acid, and deferasirox • Heavy metals—lead, mercury, and cadmium	

This constellation of findings is also referred to as Guibaud–Vainsel syndrome or marble brain disease. Other clinical features include bone fractures and growth failure. The majority of affected patients are of Arabic descent and live in North Africa and the Middle East.

What is Type 4 RTA? What are the Common Causes and Clinical Findings in Children?

Aldosterone deficiency or resistance (type 4 RTA) is due to either aldosterone deficiency or tubular resistance to the action of aldosterone. It is uncommon in children and is generally characterized by hyperkalemia and mild acidosis. In children, the most common cause of hypoaldosteronism is drugs (e.g., heparin, nonsteroidal anti-inflammatory drugs, angiotensin-converting enzyme inhibitors, trimethoprim, calcineurin) that impair aldosterone release or function. In adults, most common causes are diabetes mellitus and drugs.

Describe a Stepwise Approach to Diagnosing and Differentiating the Types of RTA

A stepwise approach to diagnosing and differentiating the types of RTA is given in **Table 4**.

Eyes/ear examination should be done in both types of RTA, as ear examination rules out deafness associated with many forms of inherited distal RTA and eye examination when indicated in proximal RTA, for example, cystine crystals (slit-lamp examination) in cystinosis (Fanconi syndrome).

TABLE 4: Stepwise approach to diagnosing and differentiating the types of RTA.

Step 1—determine anion gap (AG) in metabolic acidosis	$AG = [Na^+ - (Cl^- + HCO_3^-)]$ Corrected AG = Observed AG + 2.5 × (Routine albumin – Measured albumin) Normal AG = 8–12 ± 4–6 mEq/L when K^+ is taken into account For albumin decrease in 1 g/dL, it results in a decrease in AG by 2.5–3
Step 2—differentiate renal from extrarenal causes of acidosis	$UAG = (Na^+ + K^+) - Cl$ (representing ammonia excertion) • In extrarenal causes of normal AG acidosis, ammonia excretion increases in the tubule in form of NH_4Cl, while it remains low with renal-associated metabolic acidosis • Caveat in chronic acidosis if pH exceeds 6.5 then it measures bicarbonate ion rather ammonia as bicarbonate becomes the major anion, hence accuracy of the UAG in assessing NH_4^+ excretion decreases. In such situations, urine osmolal gap is more useful and accurate test. Urine osmolal gap = measured osmolality – calculated osmolality Calculated urine osmolality = $2[Na^+ + K^+] + UUN/2.8 + glucose/18$ Urinary NH_4^+ excretion is considered appropriately high if the gap is 100 mOsm/kg

Step 3—to ascertain the type of RTA	• Urine pH > 5.5 favors distal RTA and vice versa
	 • Caveats factors such as ammoniagenesis, urinary sodium, and infections affect urinary acidification mechanism. Excretion of low level of ammonium ion results in low urinary pH, while stimulated ammoniagenesis may have a high urine pH without having a defect in acidification. Low urinary sodium and urinary tract infection with urea-splitting organisms also can result in high urinary pH without any acidification defect
	 • To rule out false-positive high urinary pH, a modified acidification test, i.e., furosemide-fludrocortisone (FF) test should be done
	 • Tests used to differentiate RTA:
	   ○ Furosemide-fludrocortisone test
	   ○ Fractional excretion of bicarbonate >15%—favors type 2 RTA; <5% favors type 1 RTA
	   ○ Urine pCO_2 to blood pCO_2 ratio—in type 1 RTA with secretory defect (UB) CO_2 is <10, while in back leak defect of distal RTA, type II, and type IV RTA, it is >20

Step 4—in proximal channel defect, following tests to be done further to differentiate generalized form or isolated defect	• Measurement of tubular maximum reabsorption of phosphate (TmP/GFR) (Bijvoet index) is independent of serum phosphate and GFR
	   ○ Normal value is 2.8–4.4 mg/dL, which will be low in Fanconi syndrome
	   ○ TmP/GFR is a very sensitive indicator and should ideally be calculated from Bijvoet normgram
	 • In generalized aminoaciduria, proximal tubule absorbs 95–99% of amino acids. If excretion of amino acids exceeds >5%, then it is termed as generalized aminoaciduria and indicates Fanconi syndrome
	 • Tubular proteinuria—beta-2 microglobulin above upper limit suggestive of Fanconi syndrome
	 • Glucosuria threshold of glucose absorption reduced in Fanconi syndrome; hence, urinary sugar should be tested

Continued

Continued

Step 5—in distal tubule defects, tests to be done	• 24 h urine calcium—spot urine calcium/creatinine >0.2 indicates dRTA
	• USG KUB—for medullary nephrocalcinosis
	• Urinary citrate—generally reduced

(GFR: glomerular filtration rate; NH$_4$Cl: ammonium chloride; RTA: renal tubular acidosis; UAG: urine anion gap)

Describe Furosemide-fludrocortisone (FF) Test

Furosemide-fludrocortisone test is a practically feasible test for assessing the efficiency of urinary acidification mechanism. Furosemide increases delivery of sodium ion in distal tubule and, thus, enhances the urinary acidification mechanism. Mineralocorticoids support furosemide in maintaining this gradient. This test also has an important role in diagnosing incomplete distal RTA.

Prerequisite and procedure for test: It should be done with control run simultaneously and need overnight fasting and normal serum potassium.

First detect early morning urinary pH. If pH remained above 5.5, then continue the test further. Give oral furosemide dose 1 mg/kg (maximum: 40 mg) and fludrocortisone dose 0.025 mg/kg (maximum: 0.1 mg).

Allow orally during test; measure urine pH every hourly for next 4–6 hours.

Urine pH below 5.5 any time during the test is an indication for normal distal acidification mechanism and rules out type 1 RTA.

What are the Differences between Type 1 and Type 2 RTA?

The major differences between type 1 and type 2 RTA are described in **Table 5**.

What is Incomplete Distal RTA?

Incomplete distal RTA—the term "incomplete distal RTA" refers to a disorder in which there is impaired urinary acidification and an inability to reduce

TABLE 5: Differences between type 1 and type 2 renal tubular acidosis (RTA).

Parameters	Proximal RTA	Distal RTA
Pathogenesis	Defect in reabsorption of HCO$_3^-$ at proximal tubule of kidney	Defect in excretion of H$^+$ ions at distal tubule of kidney
Growth failure	Often present	Often present
Rickets–osteomalacia	Often present	Often present
Nephrocalcinosis—nephrolithiasis	Absent	Often present
Other tubular defects	Common (Fanconi syndrome)	Absent

the urine pH to 5.3 or below with an acid load exist, but net acid excretion is maintained at a rate equal to acid generation. This is achieved by an increase in ammonium excretion that offsets the reduction in titratable acid excretion caused by the high urine pH. Thus, patients with this disorder are able to maintain a normal serum bicarbonate concentration. Some patients with incomplete distal RTA progress to overt distal RTA and some have a family history of RTA.

What are the Different Presentations of Patients with Incomplete Distal RTA? When to Suspect Incomplete Distal RTA?

Patients with incomplete distal RTA have reduced urine citrate levels and may present with or develop calcium stone disease, typically calcium phosphate stones. Urine citrate excretion is increased and the frequency of stone formation is decreased by the administration of potassium citrate or potassium bicarbonate.

Otherwise unexplained osteoporosis has been described by some investigators although not confirmed by others.

Patients with recurrent calcium stones (particularly calcium phosphate stones), a normal serum bicarbonate concentration, and a urine pH that is persistently 5.5 or higher should be evaluated for incomplete distal RTA. The diagnosis should also be considered in patients with a family history of distal RTA and perhaps in those with unexplained osteoporosis. This evaluation typically includes measurement of urinary citrate excretion, which is reduced in this condition. However, a fasting morning urine pH < 5.3 and a serum potassium > 3.8 exclude nearly all patients with incomplete distal RTA.

How to Diagnose Incomplete RTA?

The diagnosis of incomplete RTA can be established by giving a single-dose oral acid load as ammonium chloride (0.1 g/kg) or a three-day modified acid load. With the single-dose acid load, serum bicarbonate concentration and urine pH are measured several times over the subsequent 6 hours, ideally at 2, 4, and 6 hours. The urine pH must be measured with a pH meter. Collection of the urine under mineral oil is not necessary. The serum bicarbonate concentration should fall by >3 mEq/L. Failure of the urine pH to fall to 5.3 or less is consistent with incomplete distal RTA.

Some patients with suspected incomplete RTA cannot tolerate the ammonium chloride because of gastric irritation, nausea, and vomiting, which occur commonly. An alternative acidification test employs the simultaneous oral administration of furosemide (40 mg) and fludrocortisone (1 mg) followed by hourly urine collections for 8 hours. Normal subjects can reduce their urine pH below 5.3 and patients with distal RTA cannot.

What are the Clinical Manifestations of Distal RTA in Infants and Children?

- Recessive form—usually presents during infancy and generally is associated with severe clinical manifestations.

  These findings include:
  - Severe hyperchloremic metabolic acidosis (serum bicarbonate levels may decrease below 10 mEq/L), moderate-to-severe hypokalemia (serum potassium ≤3.0 mEq/L), nephrocalcinosis, vomiting, dehydration, poor growth, rickets, and bilateral sensorineural hearing loss (SNHL) in some cases with mutations of the gene that encodes B1 subunit of the H-ATPase pump

- Dominant form—milder disease and presents later in life (often in adolescence and adulthood). The most common initial finding is renal stone or nephrocalcinosis. Patients typically have mild or no acidosis, mild-to-moderate hypokalemia, and, less commonly, poor growth. Bone disease is a rare finding. Mutations of the *SLC4A1* gene also are reported in some patients with hereditary spherocytosis and Southeast Asian ovalocytosis, both of which can be associated with RTA.

- Chronic kidney disease (CKD)—CKD with a glomerular filtration rate of <90 cc/min/1.73 m^2 has been reported as a complication of hereditary distal RTA. CKD presents after the pubertal growth spurt and is thought to be due to the combination of nephrocalcinosis, persistent hypokalemia, and repeated episodes of hypovolemia that results in progressive tubulointerstitial injury.

What are the Clinical Findings of Fanconi Syndrome?

It is characterized by phosphaturia resulting in hypophosphatemia, renal glucosuria, aminoaciduria, tubular proteinuria, and proximal RTA. The age of clinical presentation depends upon the underlying etiology. Clinical findings include growth failure, hypovolemia, bony abnormalities (e.g., rickets and osteomalacia), and constipation and muscle weakness due to hypokalemia.

How does Distal RTA Cause Kidney Stones?

In distal RTA, stone formation is common and most stones are calcium phosphate. The systemic metabolic acidosis leads to increased proximal tubule reabsorption of citrate, lowering urine citrate excretion. Because there is less citrate available to complex calcium, there is more calcium available to combine with phosphate or oxalate. Acidosis increases renal calcium excretion, further increasing the risk of stones. Finally, the inability to acidify urine leads to a persistent alkaline urine, which increases the amount of divalent phosphate (pK = 6.8) and, thus, the risk of calcium phosphate crystallization. CA inhibitors, such as topiramate and acetazolamide, can cause kidney stones by creating an RTA.

What is the Management of dRTA?

Correction of the acidosis with alkali is the main modality of management of RTA.

Patients with hypokalemia should be treated with potassium supplementation.

What are the Benefits of Correction of the Metabolic Acidosis in RTA?

Correction of the metabolic acidosis has a number of beneficial effects:
- Restoration of normal growth and amelioration of rickets or osteomalacia
- Diminishes renal potassium wasting and hypokalemia
- Often stabilizes or reverses nephrocalcinosis
- Reduces the frequency of calcium kidney stones and may improve osteoporosis

What is the Starting Dose of Alkali in dRTA?

Dosing of alkali therapy in adults—starting dose is 30 mEq of bicarbonate or citrate four times daily (120 mEq total per day) for patients with HCO_3^- <16 mEq/L. If the initial HCO_3^- is >16 mEq/L, starting dose is 40 mEq of bicarbonate or citrate twice daily (80 mEq total per day).

Dosing of alkali therapy in children—children usually require larger doses than adults, about 4–10 mEq/kg/day. A dose of 1 mEq/kg four times daily or 2 mEq/kg twice daily is a reasonable starting point in these patients.

How to Monitor and Adjust the Therapy?

The goal of alkali therapy is to achieve a normal serum bicarbonate concentration (22–24 mEq/L). The serum bicarbonate should be measured at approximately 1 week. The dose can then be titrated depending upon the initial response, rechecking the bicarbonate at weekly intervals until a maintenance dose is attained. This maintenance dose of bicarbonate (or citrate) is generally between 30 and 50 mEq twice daily. Once the serum chemistries have been restored to normal, the testing interval can be extended to every few months or longer. However, young children will require more frequent monitoring, since their alkali requirements will change at relatively short intervals.

Why Young Children have a Larger Alkali Requirement, Per Body Weight, than Adults?

Infants and children below the age of 6 years generate significantly larger daily acid loads (up to 10 mEq/kg) due to the deposition of alkali in the rapidly growing skeleton and a larger daily dietary caloric intake per body weight compared with older children and adults. They have a higher fixed urine pH, which results in larger ongoing bicarbonate losses. In older children, the daily acid load gradually decreases to 2–3 mEq/kg.

What are the Dosing Options for Attaining Alkali Therapy?

- Liquid sodium or potassium citrate formulations, which contain 1 mEq/mL of sodium citrate (equivalent to 1 mEq/mL of bicarbonate)
- Potassium citrate tablets, which contain 5, 10, or 15 mEq of citrate per tablet (potassium citrate with citric acid 1,100 + 334 mg)
- Sodium bicarbonate tablets, which contain either 6 mEq of bicarbonate (500 mg tablet) or 12 mEq (1,000 mg tablet). Each 84 mg of sodium bicarbonate contains 1 mEq
- Potassium bicarbonate tablets, which are available in 1,000 mg (11.9 mEq and 25 mEq sizes)
- Over-the-counter baking soda contains 27 mEq per one-half teaspoon. Dosing should be limited to one-half teaspoons at a time in order to avoid uncomfortable gastric gas formation. This is the cheapest and most readily available form of sodium bicarbonate

What are the Advantages and Disadvantages of Alkali Formulations?

Citrate may be better tolerated than bicarbonate (since there is no gastric gas formation with citrate) and is, therefore, preferred by many patients. Sodium salts will expand the extracellular fluid, which reverse volume contraction and hyperaldosteronism in some. However, sodium salts can also increase blood pressure and increase urine calcium excretion (the latter may be particularly relevant for patients who also have nephrolithiasis). Potassium salts will improve potassium depletion and hypokalemia and will generally not increase urine calcium excretion.

How to Manage Hypokalemia in dRTA?

All patients with severe or symptomatic hypokalemia should be given potassium prior to alkali therapy or at least concomitantly with bicarbonate therapy. In patients, who initially present with severe weakness or cardiac arrhythmias, intravenous potassium chloride may be required.

Correcting the metabolic acidosis with sodium-based alkali therapy typically reduces inappropriate urinary potassium losses, which often corrects the associated hypokalemia. However, some patients may have persistent hypokalemia, despite adequate correction of the volume deficit and acidosis. In such cases, potassium citrate, alone or combined with sodium citrate, must be used.

What is the Management of Proximal RTA with Fanconi Syndrome?

As in patients with distal RTA, the goal of therapy is to achieve a normal serum bicarbonate concentration (22–24 mEq/L), but this goal is often unattainable. In such cases, raising the serum bicarbonate to as near to normal as possible should be the goal.

About 10–15 mEq/kg/day of alkali is required. The alkali replacement must be given as a potassium salt (potassium citrate or potassium bicarbonate). However, in adults and older children, it may be impractical to prescribe tablets because of the high pill burden that would be required to provide adequate doses of alkali. Liquid sodium citrate/citric acid (which contains 1 mEq of citrate per mL of solution) can be used instead of or in conjunction with tablets. As an example, initial therapy could consist of 60 mL of liquid sodium citrate/citric acid two to three times daily in combination with three to four sodium bicarbonate tablets two to three times daily.

The alkali dose requirement can be reduced by diminishing the bicarbonate wasting with 12–25 mg of hydrochlorothiazide. Hydrochlorothiazide enhances bicarbonate reabsorption in the proximal tubule by reducing extracellular volume. However, thiazide diuretics will also increase urine potassium losses. A potassium-sparing diuretic (such as amiloride or spironolactone) can reduce the need for potassium supplements.

Correcting vitamin D deficiency and hypophosphatemia required in children and it will promote healing of rickets or osteomalacia.

Why High Doses of Alkali Required to Manage Proximal RTA Compared to dRTA?

Because raising the serum bicarbonate concentration will increase the filtered bicarbonate load above the proximal tubule's reduced reabsorptive capacity, it resulting in a marked bicarbonate diuresis. Thus, in contrast to the 1–2 mEq/kg/day of alkali therapy required for treatment of distal RTA, alkali doses in proximal RTA are higher. The amount of bicarbonate required will vary in different patients depending upon the extent to which the reclamation process is impaired.

Why Alkali Replacement should Give as a Potassium Salt in Proximal RTA?

The bicarbonaturia generated by alkali therapy also increases urinary potassium losses because increased sodium bicarbonate and water delivery to the distal tubule stimulate potassium secretion. As a result, an empirically determined fraction of the alkali replacement must be given as a potassium salt.

How to Monitor and Adjust the Therapy?

As with distal RTA, a reasonable monitoring schedule is to measure electrolytes (including bicarbonate, potassium, and, in patients with Fanconi syndrome, phosphate) weekly after initiating or modifying alkali therapy. Once the goal of bicarbonate level (i.e., 22–24 mEq/L) has been achieved, these measurements can be performed quarterly.

Frequent monitoring is required in young children with proximal RTA because rapid growth can lead to substantial changes in alkali requirement. If alkali therapy is modified or if other drugs are added or discontinued (e.g., thiazide or potassium-sparing diuretics), testing should be performed weekly until stable laboratory values are observed.

Proximal RTA may be a transient disorder in some children in contrast to most childhood forms of distal RTA, which are usually permanent. A rise in serum bicarbonate to above normal, thereby prompting a de-escalation of alkali therapy, is a clue that the underlying acidosis may be resolving.

How to Manage Patients with Isolated Proximal RTA?

Isolated proximal RTA is not associated with hypophosphatemia and vitamin D deficiency and, therefore, there is no need to administer phosphate or vitamin D supplements. Therapy is directed to correcting metabolic acidosis and hypokalemia as discussed above.

CONCLUSION

Renal tubular acidosis can be classified in four types. It is characterized by normal anion gap metabolic acidosis and patients have normal renal functions. Type 1 RTA can present with stunted growth, rachitic changes and failure to thrive in children. Type 2 RTA manifests with electrolyte imbalance, vomiting and dehydration. It may also lead to malnutrition and stunted growth related to loss of amino acids and glucose. Type 3 RTA has both features of distal and proximal RTA. Type 4 RTA has hyperkalemia and mild acidosis. A high index of suspicion is important in any child presenting with rickets or adult with osteomalacia. This could be presentation of distal or proximal RTA.

SUGGESTED READINGS

1. Alexander RT, Bitzan M. Renal Tubular Acidosis. Pediatr Clin North Am. 2019;66(1): 135-57.
2. Bagga A, Sinha A. Renal Tubular Acidosis. Indian J Pediatr. 2020;87(9):733-44.
3. Palmer BF, Kelepouris E, Clegg DJ. Renal Tubular Acidosis and Management Strategies: A Narrative Review. Adv Ther. 2021;38(2):949-68.
4. Pelletier J, Gbadegesin R, Staples B. Renal Tubular Acidosis. Pediatr Rev. 2017;38(11): 537-9.
5. Soares SBM, de Menezes Silva LAW, de Carvalho Mrad FC, Simões E Silva AC. Distal renal tubular acidosis: genetic causes and management. World J Pediatr. 2019;15(5):422-31.

13

CHAPTER

McCune–Albright Syndrome with Acromegaly

Kiran Kumar P, Chandar Mohan Batra

INTRODUCTION

McCune–Albright syndrome (MAS) is a noninherited rare multisystem involving syndrome. It is caused by postzygotic or sporadic or somatic mutation of *GNAS1* gene which results in constitutive activation of Gs alpha protein in the G-protein-coupled receptors (GPCR) signaling pathway. The clinical manifestations depend on the tissue which carries the mutation. Typically, MAS comprises of classic triad of precocious puberty, café-au-lait macules, and fibrous dysplasia (FD) of bone. Any two of the triad are required to diagnose MAS. Other manifestations include multiple endocrinopathies.

McCune and Albright separately described case reports of FD with extraskeletal manifestations including café-au-lait macules, precocious puberty, and hyperthyroidism. With time a number of manifestations were added to the syndrome. MAS is associated with endocrine manifestations which includes hyperthyroidism, pituitary adenomas presenting with acromegaly, prolactinomas, and Cushing's syndrome with primary adrenal hyperplasia. Bony manifestations like hypophosphatemia, osteomalacia, and rickets are also described.

CASE HISTORY

A 27-year-old man presented with complaints of increase in size of hands and legs and change in facial features since 6 years. He also had other complaints like change in voice and weight gain for past 6 years. There was no history of bone pain, fracture, visual disturbances, hearing disturbances, excessive or early facial hair growth, sexual urge, scrotal mass, gynecomastia, and galactorrhea. Patient did not have diabetes and hypertension. A birth mark on left gluteal region was present and similar birth marks were present in family members also. On examination, the patient had coarse facial features, bullous nose, macroglossia, gaps in-between the teeth, and large feet hand size with increased thickness in heel pad. Skin manifestations were excessive sebaceous secretion. Café-au-lait spots (7–8 cm) on left gluteal region were seen. Height was 184 cm and weight was 94.3 kg. There were no bony abnormalities.

Investigations

The hemogram was normal and blood biochemistry showed low calcium, low phosphate, and low vitamin D levels (5.55 ng/mL). Serum parathyroid hormone (PTH) was high (222 pg/mL). Growth hormone (GH) after 75 g of anhydrous glucose was not suppressible (15 ng/dL) and high insulin-like growth factor (IGF) level of 761 ng/mL (93–250 ng/mL) was suggestive of GH excess. Prolactin level was as 200 ng/mL. Adrenocorticotropic hormone (ACTH) level was 61 ng/mL with normal serum cortisol of 12.56 µg/dL at 8 AM and 6.49 µg/dL at 4 PM. Thyroid hormone functions showed normal thyroid-stimulating hormone (TSH) (1.32 µU/mL) with low free T4 (0.785 ng/dL). Follicle-stimulating hormone (FSH), luteinizing hormone (LH), and testosterone were normal.

Magnetic resonance imaging (MRI) sella revealed enlarged pituitary fossa with pituitary macroadenoma with sellar and suprasellar extension into optic chiasma encompassing internal carotid artery, with erosion of floor of sella seen with extension into sphenoid sinus. FD of greater and lesser wing of sphenoid bone and squamous part of temporal bone on tight side was seen (**Fig. 1**).

Perimetry revealed right temporal hemianopia and left superior quadrantanopia with normal visual acuity and normal fundus.

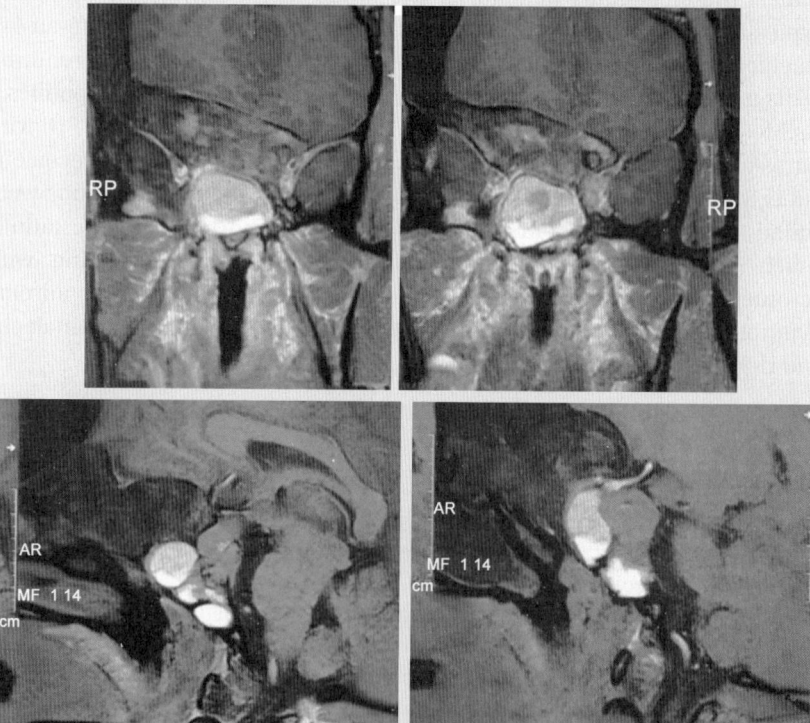

FIG. 1: MRI showing pituitary macro edema and its suprasellar and sphenoid extension. Fibrous dysplasia in sphenoid bone is also seen.

Diagnosis

With above clinical, biochemical, and imaging features our patient was diagnosed to have MAS. He had two features of the classic triad (FD and café-au-lait macules) and multiple endocrinopathies constituting acromegaly, hyperprolactinemia.

Treatment

Patient elected for definitive therapy and underwent transsphenoidal pituitary decompression under general anesthesia. Surgery was uneventful. Patient was initiated on thyroxine 75 µg daily, hydrocortisone 25 mg daily, and cabergoline 0.5 mg twice weekly postoperatively.

Outcome and Follow-up

Postoperative immediate follow-up revealed reduction in IGF1 levels to 571 (basal 761 mg/dL) and reduction in GH level to 10 ng/mL. Patient on subsequent follow-up was found symptomatically better with reduction in foot size and hand size. GH level reduced to 7.62 ng/mL, IGF level to 734 ng/mL, and prolactin to 115 ng/mL. MRI sella after 6 weeks showed reduction in tumor size (**Fig. 2**).

Further bone scan is planned to evaluate for FD and to start long-acting somatostatin LAR 20 mg monthly.

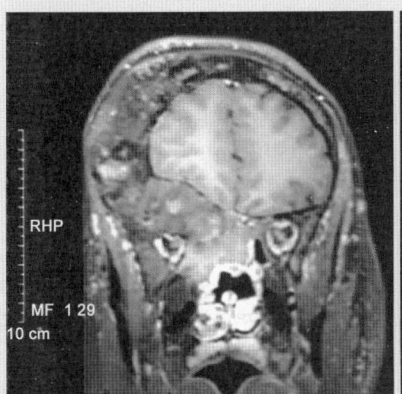
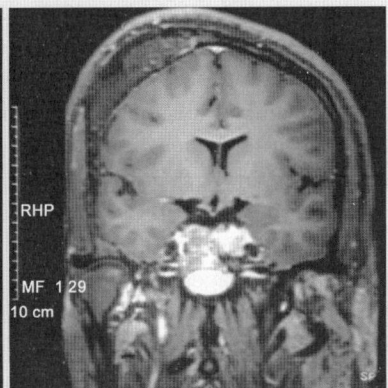
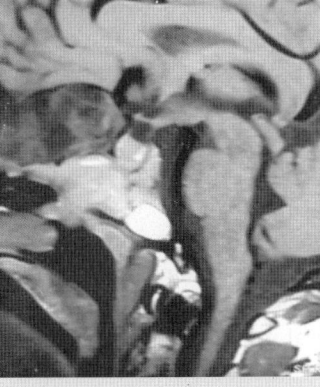

FIG. 2: Postoperative MRI showing reduction in size of tumor.

DISCUSSION

McCune–Albright syndrome is caused by early embryonic postzygotic somatic activating pathogenic variant in *GNAS* gene. Somatic *GNAS* missense mutations in MAS are known to occur in one of two amino residues Arg 201 (>95%) or Gln 227 (5%). The diagnosis is established in individuals with two or more of the classic triad, i.e., precocious puberty, café-au-lait macules, and polyostotic FD (involvement of more than one bone). If monostotic FD is found then diagnosis is established by proving *GNAS* mutation through genetic studies. The clinical features also includes the primary multiple endocrinopathies like acromegaly, hyperprolactinemia, hypercortisolemia, and hyperthyroidism.

Fibrous dysplasia exhibits mosaic pattern involving any or combination of craniofacial, axial, or appendicular skeleton with skull base and proximal femurs being most common bones. Bone pain is the common manifestation of FD, though present at any age, it is absent in childhood, occurs in adolescence, and progress through adulthood. Usually, individual bone lesions start in first decade and expand during childhood. In children, FD presents as limp, pain, or pathological fracture. In craniofacial region, it presents as painless lump or facia asymmetry and rarely with loss of vision or auditory problems due to compression of optic and auditory nerves respectively. If vertebrae is involved, it leads to scoliosis and if left untreated it results in lethal morbidity. Malignant transformation is rare but occurs in patients who were treated with radiation. Total body bone scintigraphy should be planned to identify the extent of dysplasia and the number of bones involved. Dysplastic lesions produce a phosphaturic hormone, FGF23 (Fibroblast growth factor 23), which is responsible for hypophosphatemia which may result in secondary hyperparathyroidism. Management of bone lesions includes fixation of fractures and scoliosis. Decompression of optic and auditory nerves should be done to save the visual and auditory functions. Bone pain is managed by intravenous bisphosphonates and dosing depends on symptoms rather than fixed time interval. Hypophosphatemia is managed with oral phosphorus and calcitriol.

Café-au-lait macules are common and first manifestation of MAS which can be seen shortly after birth. There is no correlation with the disease activity, location of FD with size and time of appearance of the macule. It is differentiated from neurofibromatosis by its coast of Maine border and its distribution which does not cross the midline. There are no well-defined effective treatment options.

Precocious puberty is common in girls (85%) and it is the presenting feature in majority of the patients. Recurrent ovarian cysts formation results in estrogen production and precocious puberty and sometimes patient may present with ovarian torsion. Girls are treated with aromatase inhibitor letrozole and tamoxifen a selective estrogen receptor modulator. Boys present with either unilateral or bilateral macroorchidism. Treatment of precocious puberty is not well established for boys. Spironolactone and letrozole have been tried in some cases.

Mild hyperthyroidism is common in MAS. May be either due to increased hormone production or T4 conversion to T3. GH excess is seen in 15% of individuals due to autonomous production which is associated with excessive production of prolactin. Clinical manifestation depends on the age of presentation either acromegalic features postpuberty or gigantism if presents in childhood. If GH excess is not treated, it results in expansion of craniofacial FD and lead to coarse facial features. Hypercortisolism is also seen with over production of cortisol from adrenal glands.

Methimazole is a preferred therapy but definitive treatment for hyperthyroidism is surgical resection of thyroid tissue. GH excess requires indefinite medical treatment. Definite treatment is surgical excision of total pituitary gland, but technically it is difficult and is precluded in macroadenomas and craniofacial FD. Hypercortisolism treatment have not been established because of its rarity. Medical treatment with metyrapone and ketoconazole is preferred but definitive treatment includes surgical removal of adrenal glands.

All the patients should be monitored after the surgical therapy or should be under continuous follow up to prevent complications of craniofacial FD like vision or hearing difficulties or spinal FD causing scoliosis and alteration in phosphorus levels due to continuously secreted FGF23. All the endocrinopathies are to be monitored to prevent the secondary effects of the excess hormonal secretions which is a continuing phenomenon in MAS.

CONCLUSION

Thus considering all the clinical manifestations of MAS, patients presenting with acromegaly cases should be evaluated for other hormonal excess syndromes and checked for FD and café-au-lait macules as there is no definite chronology in appearance of different manifestations of MAS.

SUGGESTED READINGS

1. Albright F, Butler AM, Hampton AO, et al. Syndrome characterized by osteitis fibrosa disseminata, areas of pigmentation and endocrine dysfunction with precocious puberty in females: Report of 5 cases. New Engl J Med. 1937;216:727-46.
2. Bhadada SK, Bhansali A, Das S, et al. Fibrous dysplasia & McCune–Albright syndrome: an experience from a tertiary care centre in north India. Indian J Med Res. 2011;133(5):504-9.
3. Boyce AM, Florenzano P, de Castro LF, et al. Fibrous dysplasia/McCune–Albright syndrome. In: Adam MP, Ardinger HH, Pagon RA, Wallace SE, Bean LJH, Stephens K, Amemiya A (Eds). GeneReviews®. Seattle (WA): University of Washington, Seattle; 2018. pp. 1993-2018.
4. Clark TJ, Tan BK, Kennedy CR. Asynchronous ovarian torsion in a patient with McCune–Albright syndrome. J Obstet Gynaecol. 2000;20:204.
5. Collins MT, Singer FR, Eugster E. McCune–Albright syndrome and the extraskeletal manifestations of fibrous dysplasia. Orphanet J Rare Dis. 2012;7 (Suppl 1):S4.
6. Diaz A, Danon M, Crawford J. McCune–Albright Syndrome and Disorders Due to Activating Mutations of GNAS1. J Pediatr Endocrinol Metabol. 2011;20(8):853-80.

7. Kelly MH, Brillante B, Collins MT. Pain in fibrous dysplasia of bone: age-related changes and the anatomical distribution of skeletal lesions. Osteoporos Int. 2008;19(1):57-63.
8. McCune DJ. Osteitis fibrosa cystica: The case of a nine-year-old girl who also exhibits precocious puberty, multiple pigmentation of the skin and hyperthyroidism. Am J Dis Child. 1936;52:743-4.
9. Salenave S, Boyce AM, Collins MT, Chanson P. Acromegaly and McCune–Albright syndrome. J Clin Endocrinol Metab. 2014;99:1955-69.

14

CHAPTER

Incidentally Detected Case of MEN1 Syndrome

Harsha Pamnani, Mohammad Asim Siddiqui

INTRODUCTION

Multiple endocrine neoplasia type 1 (MEN1/Wermer) is a rare, autosomal dominant inherited syndrome caused by mutations in the MENIN tumor suppressor gene. The diagnosis is defined clinically by the presence of two or more primary MEN1 tumors (parathyroid, anterior pituitary, and pancreatic islet). The prevalence of MEN1 is 2–3 per 100,000 and is equal among males and females. We describe the case of a patient who presented with classic history and imaging findings for MEN1.

CASE HISTORY

A 30-year-old female, mother of two children (7-year-old girl and 4-year-old boy) was referred for endocrine consultation on account for hypercalcemia when she was admitted for missed abortion. On evaluation, she was found to have serum calcium 13 mg/dL (8.6–10.2), serum albumin 4.1 g/dL, phosphorous 2.2 mg/dL (2.5–4.5), intact parathyroid hormone (iPTH) 674.6 pg/mL (15–65), and Serum TSH was 0.108 mIU/L.

Parathyroid Sestamibi Scan revealed right upper and left lower parathyroid adenoma. USG neck revealed cystic lesion in right lobe of thyroid and bilateral cystic lesions in parathyroid. Because of young age and multiple adenoma, possibility of multiple endocrine syndrome was kept. On enquiring, she had history of loss of consciousness 3 times in the past which was once found to be due to documented hypoglycemia [random blood sugar (RBS) 46 mg/dL] and it was reverted by dextrose, and at other 2 times, sugars were not measured. During hostipal stay she underwent 72 hours fast test when she developed hypoglycemia (RBS 50 mg/dL) at 10 hours. At time of hypoglycemia, serum was 30 mIU/mL, C-Peptide 1.4 nmol/L. So, the diagnosis of hyperinsulinemic hypoglycemia was made and endoscopic ultrasound was done and it was suggestive of Insulinoma. There was no history of diabetes, use of insulin, oral

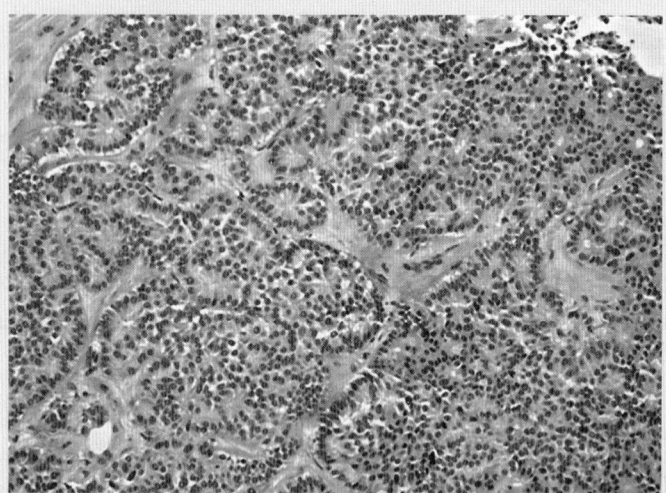

FIG. 1: Histopathology report. Well differentiated (low grade) NET of pancreas. (*For color version, see plate 6*)

hypoglycemic, herbal remedies or other prescription. MRI of brain revealed pituitary microadenoma (8.65 mm) and serum prolactin was 122.9 ng/mL (5.18–26.53).

Contrast-enhanced computed tomography (CECT) abdomen revealed multicystic lesion with calcification in tail of pancreas. Bilateral renal cysts were also seen. Endoscopic fine-needle aspiration cytology (FNAC) from solid mass in retroperitoneum revealed pancreatic neuroendocrine tumor (NET) grade 2 (**Fig. 1**), Ki67—8%. Serum cortisol and 24 hours urinary metanephrines and normetanephrines were normal. 5-hydroxyindoleacetic acid (5-HIAA) and chromogranin were normal. DOTA PET revealed pancreatic tail lesion 24 × 23 mm and 22 × 20 mm. Parathyroid uptake was seen and two lesions were noted in relation to left adrenal.

Total parathyroidectomy and right hemithyroidectomy with autotransplantation of parathyroid gland in left brachioradialis muscle was done. Immediately after surgery, postoperative PTH fell within normal range. The histopathological report was parathyroid hyperplasia and hyperplastic nodule in thyroid.

Distal pancreaticosplenectomy + left adrenalectomy + cholecystectomy were done after 4 weeks of the first surgery. Biopsy revealed low-grade NET, adrenal cortical adenoma, normal gallbladder, and omentum and spleen mixed red pulp congestion. There was no episode of hypoglycemia documented in the last 6 months on follow-up.

After two and half months of surgery, patient's prolactin level was still elevated and she was started on cabergoline with normalization of prolactin levels. Currently, the patient is doing well and is under regular follow-up.

DISCUSSION

The first case of MEN1 was published by Erdheim in 1903. In 1953, Underdahl et al. introduce the term "multiple endocrine adenomas" and reported the first familial occurrence of this syndrome. In 1954, Wermer postulated that this syndrome is caused by mutation in a single gene and inherited in an autosomal dominant.

The *MEN1* gene is a classic tumor suppressor gene which encodes the menin protein. The site of the "*MEN1* gene" is region on the long arm of chromosome 11 (11q13). Menin is a ubiquitous nuclear protein involved in regulation of gene transcription. Menin is a suppressor of the expression of the telomerase gene hTERT. Possibly, inactivation of menin could lead to cell immortalization by telomerase expression, which could allow a cell to develop into a tumor cell.

Basis for a diagnosis of MEN1 in individuals. A diagnosis of MEN1 may be established in an individual by one of three criteria (**Flowchart 1**).

Direct DNA sequence analysis remains the method of choice in most clinical diagnostic laboratories and is considered as the "gold standard". Complete *MEN1* gene sequencing is the best method and positive in 70–90% of typical MEN1 cases. Multiplex ligation-dependent probe amplification (MLPA) assay is a recent development for detection of large deletions occurring in 4% of MEN1 cases. Some families may harbor mutations in regulatory sequences, regions which are not investigated on a routine basis, so no *MEN1* gene germline mutation can be found, even if testing for gross deletions is included.

Several families with a MEN1-like disorder have germline mutations in *AIP* (aryl hydrocarbon receptor interacting protein) gene predisposing to pituitary adenoma and mutations of the *CDKN1B* (p27Kip1) gene in patients with MEN4. CDKN1A, CDKN2B, and CDKN2C may also be involved. Mutational analysis of the AIP and *CDKN1B* genes should be considered in *MEN1* gene mutation negative families.

Primary hyperparathyroidism is the most common (90%) and first detected endocrinopathy presenting with mild hypercalcemia and rarely

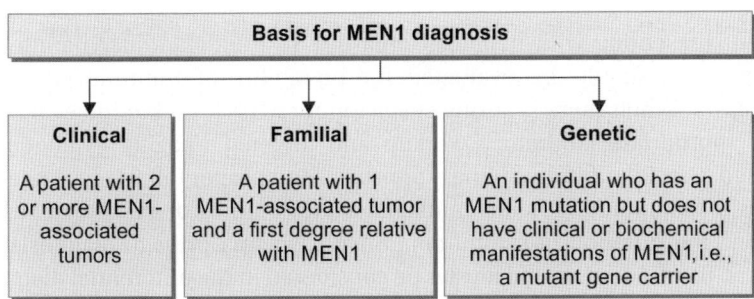

FLOWCHART 1: Basis of multiple endocrine neoplasia type 1 (MEN1) diagnosis.

severe hypercalcemia in MEN1. The age of onset in primary hyperparathyroidism is earlier as compared to that in sporadic hyperparathyroidism (20–25 years vs. 55 years).

Greater reduction in bone mineral density may be found and male/female ratio is 1:1 in MEN1 while it is 1:3 in sporadic cases. Removal of all four parathyroids with transplantation of one-half a gland into the forearm with bilateral transcervical thymectomy is the procedure of choice for MEN1-related hyperparathyroidism.

Pancreatic NETs develop in about 55% of MEN1 patients. Multicentric microadenomas are present in 90% of MEN1 patients. Most of them are nonfunctional. Among functional tumors, gastrinoma is more common than insulinoma.

Pituitary tumors in MEN1 are larger in size and more aggressive than sporadic tumors. Prolactinoma is the most frequently occurring pituitary tumor in MEN1. MEN1 must be considered in all children with tumors of the pituitary gland.

Periodic clinical monitoring should be done in MEN1 patients, *MEN1* gene germline mutation carriers, and MEN1-suspected patients without a confirmed mutation.

Periodical screening includes:
- *From the age of 5, biannual clinical examination*: Laboratory investigation including measurement in blood of ionized calcium, chloride, phosphate, parathyroid hormone, glucose, insulin, c-peptide, glucagon, gastrin, pancreatic polypeptide, prolactin, insulin-like growth factor 1, platelet serotonin, and chromogranin A
- *From the age of 15, radiological screening once every 2 years (but no gamma radiation)*: MRI of the upper abdomen, MRI of the pituitary with gadolinium contrast, and MRI of the mediastinum in males
- Endoscopic ultrasonography (EUS) of the upper abdomen may permit earlier detection of pancreatic pathology

Genetic study of MEN1 was not performed in our case because of the presence of insulinoma, parathyroid adenoma, and pituitary adenoma.

CONCLUSION

Patient presenting with hypercalcemia due to multiglandular parathyroid involvement should be evaluated for possibility of multiple endocrine neoplasm. When there is strong suspicion for MEN1, endocrine evaluation with appropriate laboratory workup and targeted imaging evaluation is needed. Careful multidisciplinary approach and proper follow-up is needed. Cases of insulinoma remains undiagnosed for months or even years. In our patient, the duration of symptoms of hypoglycemia prior to diagnosis was 3 years. Insulinoma should always be considered in the differential diagnosis of all cases of nondiabetic hypoglycemia, since early detection and timely management could be lifesaving. Pedigree studies have to be performed to detect second and third grade family members at risk. Gastrinomas and other NETs have malignant potential. Periodic clinical monitoring makes pre-symptomatic detection and treatment of MEN1-associated tumors possible.

SUGGESTED READINGS

1. Erdheim J. Zur normalen und pathologischen Histologie der Glandula Thyreoidea, Para-thyreoidea und Hypophysis. Beitr Pathol Anat. 1903;33:158-263.
2. Georgitsi M, Raitila A, Karhu A, et al. Molecular diagnosis of pituitary adenoma predisposition caused by aryl hydrocarbon receptor-interacting protein gene mutations. Proc Natl Acad Sci USA. 2007;104(10):4101-5.
3. Kouvaraki MA, Shapiro SE, Cote GJ, et al. Management of pancreatic endocrine tumors in Multiple Endocrine Neoplasia Type 1. World J Surg. 2006;30(5):643-53.
4. Lemos MC, Thakker RV. Multiple endocrine neoplasia type 1 (MEN1): analysis of 1336 mutations reported in the first decade following identification of the gene. Hum Mutat. 2008;29(1):22-32.
5. Pieterman CR, Vriens MR, Dreijerink KM, et al. Care for patients with multiple endocrine neoplasia type 1: the current evidence base. Fam Cancer. 2011;10(1):157-71.
6. Rix M, Hertel NT, Nielsen FC, et al. Cushing's disease in childhood as the first manifestation of multiple endocrine neoplasia syndrome type 1. Europ J Endocr. 2004;15(1):709-15.
7. Thakker RV, Newey PJ, Walls GV, et al; Endocrine Society. Clinical Practice Guidelines for Multiple Endocrine Neoplasia Type 1 (MEN1). J Clin Endocrinol Metab. 2012;97(9):2990-3011.
8. Wermer P. Genetic aspects of adenomatosis of endocrine glands. Am J Med Sci. 1954;16(3):363-71.

15
CHAPTER

Young Hypertension Secondary to Primary Hyperaldosteronism

Monika Goyal, Chandar Mohan Batra

INTRODUCTION

Hypertension is primarily considered a disease of old age but studies done in USA show that 1 in 3 young adults have hypertension. Similarly as per an article published in European Society of Cardiology 1 in every 5 young adults in India have high blood pressure (BP) equating to around 80 million people. About 90% of these have essential hypertension but rest 10% have secondary hypertension. Younger the patient more is the probability of them having secondary hypertension. It is important to diagnose these secondary causes of hypertension as they are potentially correctable and have significant effect on reducing mortality. The causes of secondary hypertension include renal parenchymal disease, coarctation of aorta, fibromuscular disease, endocrinological causes including Cushing disease, pheochromocytoma, primary hyperaldosteronism, and other rare causes including obstructive sleep apnea. The diagnosis of these disorder can be suggested by specific history of pedal edema, flushing, palpitations (pheochromocytoma), weight gain, hirsutism (Cushing's syndrome), or examination finding of a classical murmur in coarctation in aorta, purplish striae in Cushing's, or hypokalemia in primary hyperaldosteronism. Management depends on underlying cause of hypertension. We are discussing a case of 34-year-old young hypertensive diagnosed to be having primary hyperaldosteronism and his management in our hospital.

CASE HISTORY

We are discussing a case report of a 34-year-old male patient who presented to our OPD with complaints of uncontrolled hypertension. Patient was diagnosed to be hypertensive 3 years back, when he visited a hospital in Bangkok for the complaints of muscle cramps. His BP recorded was 180/110 mm Hg in the Bangkok hospital. He was given antihypertensive drugs and oral potassium. He was also told about some abdominal tumor, but did not have any records when he visited our hospital. He was on two antihypertensive tablets—losartan 50 mg twice a day and nifedipine 20 mg per oral three times a day. He did not give any history suggestive of renal disease, heart disease, or obstructive sleep apnea (OSA). On examination, his pulse was 80 bpm, regular and equally palpable in all four limbs with no radiofemoral delay. His BP was 160/110 mm Hg in all four limbs without any postural drop. His systemic examination was normal. No renal bruit was present. On investigation, his serum creatinine was 0.8 mg/dL, serum urea 24 mg/dL, sodium 145 mEq/L, potassium 4.2 mEq/L. His serum cortisol was 16.81 µg/dL at 8 AM, 9.77 µg/dL at 4 PM; 24-hour urinary epinephrine was 11.15 µg/24 h (4–20); norepinephrine was 43.38 µg/24 h (23–105); and dopamine was 407 µg/24 h (62–446). Serum dehydroepiandrosterone sulfate (DHEAS) was 236.3 µg/dL (139.7–484.4). Plasma aldosterone was 45.5 ng/dL, plasma renin activity 0.01 ng/mL/h, plasma aldosterone-to-renin ratio (ARR) was 4,550 ng/dL/ng/mL/h. Magnetic resonance imaging (MRI) of abdomen was done and is suggestive of well-defined nodular lesion in right adrenal gland arising from its anterior limb measuring around 1.2 × 1.4 cm in size, no area of necrosis and hemorrhage were seen with in the tumor. Left adrenal gland was normal. We finally made a diagnosis of primary hyperaldosteronism (Conn's syndrome) due to right adrenal adenoma. We did not do further confirmatory test since he was a young patient diagnosed with hypertension at the age of 31 years, had accelerated hypertension with BP at baseline being 180/110 mm Hg, had history of hypokalemia with high plasma aldosterone and suppressed renin, high ARR, and MRI abdomen suggestive of unilateral adenoma. We advised the patient for adrenal venous sampling (AVS) and regarding further need of adrenalectomy. But patient refused for the same. He was started on tablet spironolactone 25 mg twice a day. Patient is doing well since then. His BP is maintaining around 130/90 mm Hg with no further episode of hypokalemia.

DISCUSSION

Young hypertension is defined as hypertension in people below the age group of 40 years. Even though 90% of these patients have essential hypertension, approximately 5–10% of adult have secondary causes. Factors that point toward secondary causes are younger age group, rapid onset, accelerated hypertension, and resistant hypertension. The cause is variable according to age. Renal artery stenosis is more common in younger age group while primary hyperaldosteronism is more common in adult population. It is important to recognize them since many of these diseases are amenable to treatment. Not treating this disease puts these patients at higher risk of cardiovascular mortality.

Among secondary causes of hypertension one of the important cause of hypertension in young adult is primary hyperaldosteronism. It is an endocrine disorder characterized by excessive aldosterone production inappropriately high for sodium status, relatively autonomous of the major regulators of secretion (angiotensin II, plasma potassium concentration), and nonsuppressible by sodium loading.

Aldosterone is a steroid hormone secreted by zona glomerulosa of adrenal gland. Its secretion is regulated mainly by three factors angiotensin II, potassium, and adrenocorticotropic hormone (ACTH); all three of them increase aldosterone while dopamine, atrial natriuretic peptide, and heparin inhibit aldosterone secretion. The secretion of angiotensin is in turn regulated by renin.

About 50–70% aldosterone circulating is albumin bound or weakly bound to corticosteroid-binding globulin while rest of 30–50% is available freely for action. It has a short half-life of 15–20 minutes, and is then inactivated in liver to tetrahydroaldosterone. Its main function is to maintain extracellular volume and potassium homeostasis. It acts primarily by binding to mineralocorticoid receptor (MR) in cytosol of epithelial cell principally in the kidney's distal nephron, colon, and hippocampus where it is present in the highest concentration, while lower levels are seen in heart and gastrointestinal tract. Its action on MR increases apical membrane sodium channel expression and increases sodium ion transport across cell membrane, causing volume expansion and hypertension. Also due to sodium absorption, intraluminal negativity increases, leading to increased tubular cell potassium excretion and interstitial cell hydrogen ion secretion leading to hypokalemia and metabolic alkalosis in patient with primary hyperaldosteronism.

It also has additional nonclassical action, i.e., increasing expression of several collagen genes, gene-controlling tissue growth, and gene-mediating inflammation resulting in increase in microangiopathy, necrosis, and fibrosis at various tissue such as heart, vasculature, and kidney.

Primary hyperaldosteronism was first described in 1955 by Dr Jerome W Conn. It is responsible for 5–10% of total cases of hypertension making it a public health problem. Although hypokalemia considered its sine qua non of primary hyperaldosteronism, it is seen only in 10–40% of patients. It is usually caused by either aldosterone-producing adenoma (APA) (30%) and bilateral idiopathic hyperaldosteronism (60%); other rare causes include primary unilateral adrenal hyperplasia (UAH), aldosterone-producing adrenocortical carcinoma, familial hyperaldosteronism (FH) type I, II, III and rarely ectopic APA or carcinoma.

Patients generally present between third to fifth decade of life with accelerated hypertension. The endocrine society clinical practice guidelines suggest that primary hyperaldosteronism should be suspected in patients with sustained BP above 150/100 mm Hg on each of three measurements obtained on different days, with hypertension (BP >140/90 mm Hg) resistant to three conventional antihypertensive drugs (including a diuretic), or controlled BP (<140/90 mm Hg) on four or more antihypertensive drugs; hypertension and spontaneous or diuretic-induced hypokalemia, hypertension and adrenal incidentaloma, hypertension and sleep apnea; hypertension and a family history of early onset hypertension or cerebrovascular accident at a young age (<40 years), and all hypertensive first-degree relatives of patients with primary hyperaldosteronism.

Occasionally, patient can also present with symptoms of marked hypokalemia, may have muscle weakness, cramping, palpitation, and periodic paralysis. Periodic paralysis is rare in Caucasians but found mainly in Asians. Rarely, they may present with tetany due to decreased ionized calcium with marked hypokalemic alkalosis. They may also have polyuria and nocturia due to hypokalemia-induced renal concentrating defect. Edema is not seen usually due to mineralocorticoid escape phenomenon. Patients with long-standing hyperaldosteronism may develop chronic kidney disease and left ventricular hypertrophy, myocardial infarction, stroke, and arrhythmias.

Once suspected of primary hyperaldosteronism, these patient should undergo screening test, i.e., paired measurement of plasma aldosterone concentration and plasma renin activity (PAC/PRA) ratio in a random ambulatory morning blood sample preferable between 8 AM to 10 AM as a screening test. Hypokalemia reduces the secretion of aldosterone and it is optimal to restore normokalemia before performing diagnostic tests. Various antihypertensive drugs can affect the PAC, PRA value, and ARR ratio and according these drugs need to be stopped or switched over to drugs that have minimal effect of renin aldosterone system. The endocrine society clinical practice guideline gives recommendation as given in **Box 1**.

BOX 1 | **Preparation of patient prior to doing ARR.**

- Correct hypokalemia
- Liberal sodium intake
- Withdraw agents that markedly affect the ARR for at least 4 weeks:
  - Spironolactone, eplerenone, amiloride, and triamterene
  - Potassium-wasting diuretics
  - Products derived from licorice root (e.g., confectionary licorice and chewing tobacco)
- If the results of ARR after discontinuation of the above agents are not diagnostic, and if hypertension can be controlled with relatively noninterfering medications, withdraw other medications that may affect the ARR for at least 2 weeks, such as:
  - β-adrenergic blockers, central 2 agonists (e.g., clonidine and α-methyldopa), and nonsteroidal anti-inflammatory drugs
  - Angiotensin-converting enzyme inhibitors, angiotensin receptor blockers, renin inhibitors, and dihydropyridine calcium channel antagonists
- If necessary continue other antihypertensive medications that have lesser effects on the ARR [e.g., verapamil slow-release, hydralazine (with verapamil slow-release, to avoid reflex tachycardia), prazosin, doxazosin, and terazosin]
- Establish OC and HRT status that affect ARR ratio

Conditions for blood collection:
- Collect blood mid-morning, after the patient has been up (sitting, standing, or walking) for at least 2 h and seated for 5–15 min
- Collect blood carefully, avoiding stasis and hemolysis
- Maintain sample at room temperature (and not on ice, as this will promote conversion of inactive to active renin) during delivery to laboratory and prior to centrifugation and rapid freezing of plasma component pending assay

(ARR: aldosterone–to–renin ratio; OC: oral contraceptive; HRT: hormone replacement therapy)

A high PAC/PRA ratio is a positive screening test result, a finding that warrants further testing. Most studies show that a PAC/PRA ratio of >20, a plasma aldosterone >15 ng/dL, and a low plasma renin activity are highly suggestive of primary hyperaldosteronism.

An increased PAC/PRA itself is not diagnostic of primary hyperaldosteronism and should be confirmed by confirmatory test, i.e., aldosterone suppression test. The different tests that can be performed include oral sodium loading test, intravenous saline infusion test, and fludrocortisone suppression test. Oral sodium loading test is done by increasing their sodium intake to 200 mmol (6 g)/day for 3 days, verified by 24-hour urine sodium content along with potassium supplement to maintain potassium in normal range. Urinary aldosterone is measured in the 24-hour urine collection from the morning of day 3 to the morning of day 4. Primary aldosteronism (PA) is unlikely if urinary aldosterone is <10 g/24 h (28 nmol/day) in the absence of renal disease. Elevated urinary aldosterone excretion [>12 g/24 h (>33 nmol/day)] makes PA highly likely.

For saline infusion test patient should stay recumbent for at least 1 hour before and during the infusion of 2 liters of 0.9% intravenous (IV) saline over 4 hour starting at 8–9.30 AM. Blood samples for renin, aldosterone, cortisol, and plasma potassium are drawn at time zero and after 4 hours, with BP and heart rate monitored throughout the test. Postinfusion plasma aldosterone levels <5 ng/ dL (140 pmol/L) make the diagnosis of PA unlikely, whereas levels >10 ng/dL (280 nmol/L) are a sign of very probable PA. Values between 5 ng/dL and 10 ng/dL are indeterminate, although a cutoff of 6.8 ng/dL (190 pmol/L) has been found to offer the best trade-off between sensitivity and specificity.

Last test that can be done is fludrocortisone suppression test. Patients receive 0.1 mg oral fludrocortisone every 6 hours for 4 days, together with slow-release KCl supplements (every 6 h at doses sufficient to keep plasma K^+, measured four times a day, close to 4.0 mmol/L), slow-release NaCl supplements (30 mmol three times daily with meals), and sufficient dietary salt to maintain a urinary sodium excretion rate of at least 3 mmol/kg body weight. On day 4, plasma aldosterone and PRA are measured at 10 AM with the patient in the seated posture, and plasma cortisol is measured at 7 and 10 AM. Upright plasma aldosterone >6 ng/dL (170 nmol/L) on day 4 at 10 AM confirms PA, provided PRA is <1 ng/mL/h and plasma cortisol concentration is lower than the value obtained at 7 AM to exclude a confounding ACTH effect. These tests should not be performed in patients with severe uncontrolled hypertension, renal insufficiency, cardiac arrhythmia, or severe hypokalemia.

In a biochemically confirmed case of primary hyperaldosteronism further radiological tests are done which help to determine therapeutic approach. Investigations done are computed tomography (CT) of adrenals and AVS. First investigation to be done is adrenal CT. It serves two purposes, i.e., to subtype the tumor and to exclude any large mass that may represent adrenocortical carcinoma. In a study of 203 patient, it was found that isolated adrenal CT was accurate only in 53% of patients. CT may appear normal or may incidentally show bilateral nodularity in a patient with small APA. A non-functioning unilateral adenoma are not uncommon especially in a patient older than 40 years of age. In a systematic review of 38 studies involving 950 patients with PA, adrenal CT/MRI results did not agree with the findings from AVS in 359 patients (38%); based on CT/MRI, 19% of the 950 patients would have undergone noncurative surgery, and 19% would have been offered medical therapy instead of curative adrenalectomy. Therefore, AVS is essential to direct appropriate therapy in patients with PA who have a high probability of APA and are seeking a potential surgical cure.

It has been recommended when surgical treatment is possible or desired by the patients, an invasive radiologist should use AVS to make a distinction between unilateral and bilateral adrenal disease. Except in case of younger patient age <35 years of age with spontaneous hypokalemia, marked aldosterone excess and unilateral adrenal lesion with radiological features consistent with a cortical adenoma on adrenal CT scan may not need AVS before proceedings to unilateral adrenalectomy. The sensitivity and specificity of AVS is 95% and 100%, respectively to detect unilateral aldosterone excess and is superior to adrenal CT with sensitivity and specificity of 78% and 75%, respectively. AVS is a difficult invasive procedure. Cannulating right adrenal vein is more difficult than due to its smaller diameter. The cannulating accuracy improves to 90–96% in experienced hands. Simultaneous measurement of cortisol in adrenal vein and calculating cortisol corrected ratio improved the accuracy of catheter placement. The AVS can be done by three protocols: (1) Unstimulated sequential or simultaneous bilateral AVS; (2) Unstimulated sequential or simultaneous bilateral AVS followed by bolus cosyntropin-stimulated sequential or simultaneous AVS; and (3) Continuous cosyntropin infusion with sequential bilateral AVS. Bilateral AVS is difficult to perform and not performed at most of the centers. With continuous cosyntropin administration the cutoff of the cortisol-corrected aldosterone ratio from high-side to low-side of more than 4 indicates unilateral aldosterone excess; a ratio of <3:1 is suggestive of bilateral aldosterone hypersecretion. With these cutoffs, AVS for detecting unilateral aldosterone hypersecretion (APA or UAH) has a sensitivity of 95% and specificity of 100%. Patients with lateralization ratios between 3:1 and 4:1 may have either unilateral or bilateral disease, and the AVS results must be cautiously interpreted in conjunction with the clinical setting, CT scan, ancillary tests, and if possible, repeat AVS.

In the absence of cosyntropin stimulation cortisol-corrected aldosterone lateralization ratio (high to low side) is more than 2:1 and consistent with unilateral disease. Other groups rely primarily on comparing the adrenal vein aldosterone-cortisol ratios to those in a simultaneously collected peripheral venous sample. When the aldosterone-cortisol ratio from an adrenal vein is significantly (usually at least 2.5 times) greater than that of the peripheral

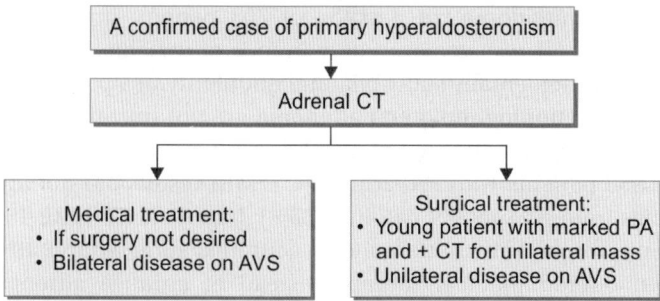

(AVS: adrenal venous sampling; PA: primary aldosteronism)

FLOWCHART 1: Algorithm to approach a case of primary hyperaldosteronism.

vein (cubital fossa or inferior vena cava), and the aldosterone-cortisol ratio in the contralateral adrenal vein is no higher than peripheral (indicating contralateral suppression), this is interpreted as showing lateralization, an indication that unilateral adrenalectomy should cure or improve the hypertension (**Flowchart 1**).

Management of PA can be done either surgically or medically. Surgery, laparoscopic unilateral adrenalectomy, is recommended in patients with documented unilateral PA (i.e., APA or UAH) except in those unable or unwilling to undergo surgery. Prior to surgery both hypertension and hypokalemia should be well controlled before patients undergo surgery. After the surgery, potassium supplementation is withdrawn on postoperative day 1, spironolactone is discontinued, and antihypertensive therapy is reduced. Postoperative intravenous fluids should be normal saline without potassium chloride unless serum potassium levels remain very low (i.e., 3.0 mmol/L); along with generous sodium intake to avoid postoperative hyperkalemia due to chronic contralateral adrenal suppression. Plasma aldosterone and renin activity levels shortly are measured 2 days after surgery as an early indication of biochemical response, although renin levels may not fall immediately. Persistent hypoaldosteronism requiring mineralocorticoid replacement therapy (fludrocortisone) may occur in up to 5% of adrenalectomized patients. Surgery normalizes serum potassium concentrations in nearly 100% of patients postoperatively. While BP control improves in 100% but hypertension is cured (defined as BP 140/90 mm Hg without the aid of antihypertensive drugs) in about 50%. Factors predisposing to persistent hypertension are having more than one first-degree relative with hypertension, use of two more antihypertensive preoperatively, old age, increased creatinine, duration of hypertension, and mostly due to co-existent primary hypertension. Surgery also improves quality of life, reduces morbidity or mortality, and reverses the increase in carotid intima-media thickness and arterial stiffness.

In patients with PA due to bilateral adrenal disease, or those with unilateral adrenal disease but not willing for surgery or unable to undergo surgery, medical treatment is recommended with an MR antagonist. Spironolactone is used as the primary agent, with eplerenone as an alternative. Sodium should be restricted diet <100 mEq of sodium per day, ideal body weight should be maintained, tobacco should be avoided.

Spironolactone is the first drug of choice. Started in the dose of 12.5, 25 mg on to maximum of 400 mg/day to achieve normal serum potassium without aid of potassium supplement. Hypokalemia responds promptly while hypertension takes 4–8 weeks. It reduces mean systolic BP by 25% and diastolic BP by 22%. On therapy, potassium and creatinine is monitored frequently during the first 4–6 week of therapy. Side effect includes anti-testosterone effect leading to painful gynecomastia, erectile dysfunction, and decreased libido while progesterone agonist activity is responsible for menstrual irregularity in women.

Eplerenone is a newer, selective MR antagonist without antiandrogen and progesterone agonist effects. The starting dose for eplerenone is 25 mg twice daily. Eplerenone is used as second-line agent. It is a steroid-based antimineralocorticoid agent that act as a competitive and selective MR antagonist. Its 9–11 epoxide group has reduced marked progestational and antiandrogenic actions and has 0.1% affinity to androgen receptor and <1% binding to progesterone receptor. Eplerenone causes less gynecomastia and female mastodynia but is less effective in BP control. Started with 25 mg BD, given to a maximum of 100 mg/day. Side effects like dizziness, headache, fatigue, diarrhea, hypertriglyceridemia, and elevated liver enzymes may be seen. If patient do not respond to these drugs it is mainly because of volume overload and do well with addition of thiazides.

Other drugs that can be used are epithelial sodium channel antagonists amiloride and triamterene. Amiloride has been the more studied as a mode of treatment for PA. Calcium channel blockers, angiotensin-converting enzyme inhibitors, and angiotensin receptor blocker are used as add-on therapy.

There are few familial cause of PA. FH-1 [glucocorticoid-remediable aldosteronism (GRA)] is inherited in an autosomal dominant fashion and is responsible for 1% of cases of PA. It occurs due to fusion of the promoter region of the gene for *CYP11B1* and the coding sequences of *CYP11B2*, resulting in a *CYP11B1/CYP11B2* chimeric gene, putting aldosterone under ACTH regulation. Studies suggest a high pretest probability for GRA in children or young adults with severe or resistant hypertension and a positive family history of early onset hypertension (<20 years of age) and/or premature hemorrhagic stroke. Genetic testing by either Southern blot or long polymerase chain reaction (PCR) techniques for the underlying hybrid *CYP11B1/CYP11B2* mutation is sensitive and specific for GRA and should replace indirect testing (e.g., urinary levels of 18-oxocortisol and 18-hydroxy-cortisol, or dexamethasone suppression testing), both of which may be misleading.

In patients with GRA, we recommend administering the lowest dose of glucocorticoid to lower ACTH and thus normalize BP and potassium levels as the first-line treatment. In addition, if BP fails to normalize with glucocorticoid alone, an MR antagonist may be added (eplerenone is preferred in children). For children, the glucocorticoid dosage should be adjusted for age and body weight, and BP targets should be determined from age- and gender-specific published normative data. The glucocorticoid should be taken at bedtime. The dose of dexamethasone is 0.125–0.25 mg/day.

In case of children, short-acting steroids like hisone or prednisolone may be given at bed time according to body surface area to maintain BP in age specific ranges. Careful attention should be given to growth retardation due to overtreatment. Steroids may even have role in normotensive GRA patients.

Familial hyperaldosteronism type II (FH-II) is an autosomal dominant disorder, genetically heterogeneous, and is more common than FH-I, accounting for at least 7% of patients with PA in one series, but its true prevalence is unknown. The molecular basis for FH-II is unclear, although several linkage analyses have shown an association with chromosomal region 7p22. FH-III was first described in a family characterized by severe hypertension in early childhood associated with hyperaldosteronism, hypokalemia, and resistance to antihypertensive therapy, requiring bilateral adrenalectomy. A mutation was found in the *KCNJ5* gene encoding the potassium channel Kir 3.4 (potassium inwardly rectifying channel, subfamily 1, member 5), resulting in increased sodium conductance and cell depolarization. In very young patients with PA, it is suggested to test for germline mutations in *KCNJ5* causing FH-III.

CONCLUSION

To conclude, need to recognize primary hyperaldosteronism as a public health problem with incidence of 5–10% and therefore broaden our indications for screening, and to include subjects with sustained BP elevation above 150 mm Hg (systolic) and/or 100 mm Hg (diastolic). Once suspected a paired sample of plasma aldosterone and plasma renin activity with ARR should be send as a screening testing. For patent with high ARR further confirmatory testing and subtyping is done to decide management. Timely diagnosis and treatment of PA, reduces cardiovascular and renal damage.

SUGGESTED READINGS

1. Ahmed AH, Cowley D, Wolley M, et al. Seated saline suppression testing for the diagnosis of primary aldosteronism: a preliminary study. J Clin Endocrinol Metab. 2014;99:2745-53.
2. Fardella CE, Pinto M, Mossol, et al. Genetic study of patients with dexamethasone-suppressible aldosteronism without the chimeric CYP11B1/CYP11B2 gene. J Clin Endocrinol Metab. 2001;86:4805-7.
3. Funder JW, Carey RM, Fardella C, et al. Case detection, diagnosis, and treatment of patients with primary aldosteronism: an Endocrine Society clinical practice guideline. J Clin Endocrinol Metab. 2008;93:3266-81.

4. Funder JW, Carey RM, Mantero F, et al. The management of primary aldosteronism: case detection, diagnosis, and treatment: an endocrine society clinical practice guideline. J Clin Endocrinol Metab. 2016;101(5):1889-916.

5. Funder JW. The nongenomic actions of aldosterone. Endocr Rev. 2005;26:313-21.

6. Hiramatsu K, Yamada T, Yukimura Y, et al. A screening test to identify aldosterone-producing adenoma by measuring plasma renin activity. Results in hypertensive patients. Arch Intern Med. 1981;141:1589-93.

7. Iwakura Y, Morimoto R, Kudo M, et al. Predictors of decreasing glomerular filtration rate and prevalence of chronic kidney disease after treatment of primary aldosteronism: renal outcome of 213 cases. J Clin Endocrinol Metab. 2014;99:1593-8.

8. Jonsson JR, Klemm SA, Tunny TJ, et al. A new genetic test for familial hyperaldosteronism type I aids in the detection of curable hypertension. Biochem Biophys Res Comm. 1995;207:565-71.

9. Kempers MJ, Lenders JW, van Outheusden L, et al. Systematic review: diagnostic procedures to differentiate unilateral from bilateral adrenal abnormality in primary aldosteronism. Ann Intern Med. 2009;151:329-37.

10. Ma JT, Wang C, Lam KS, et al. Fifty cases of primary hyperaldosteronism in Hong Kong Chinese with a high frequency of periodic paralysis. Evaluation of techniques for tumour localisation. Q J Med. 1986;61:1021-37.

11. Melmed S, Polonsky KS, Larsen RP, Kronenberg MK (Eds). Williams Textbook of Endocrinology, 13th edition. Elsevier Health Sciences; 2015.

12. Mulatero P, Stowasser M, Loh KC, et al. Increased diagnosis of primary aldosteronism, including surgically correctable forms, in centers from five continents. J Clin Endocrinol Metab. 2004;89:1045-50.

13. Piaditis G, Markou A, Papanastasiou L, et al. Progress in primary aldosteronism: a review of the prevalence of primary aldosteronism in pre-hypertension and hypertension. Eur J Endocrinol. 2015;172(5):R191-R203.

14. Rossi GP, Auchus RJ, Brown M, et al. An expert consensus statement on use of adrenal vein sampling for the subtyping of primary aldosteronism. Hypertension. 2014;63:151-60.

15. Rossi GP, Sacchetto A, Chiesura-Corona M, et al. Identification of the etiology of primary aldosteronism with adrenal vein sampling in patients with equivocal computed tomography and magnetic resonance findings: results in 104 consecutive cases. J Clin Endocrinol Metab. 2001;86:1083-90.

16. Rossi GP, Sacchetto A, Visentin P, et al. Changes in left ventricular anatomy and function in hypertension and primary aldosteronism. Hypertension. 1996;27:1039-45.

17. Stowasser M. Update in primary aldosteronism. J Clin Endocrinol Metab. 2015;100:1-10.

18. Tanabe A, Naruse M, Naruse K, et al. Left ventricular hypertrophy is more prominent in patients with primary aldosteronism than inpatients with other types of secondary hypertension. Hypertens Res. 1997;20:85-90.

19. Viera AJ, Neutze D. Diagnosis of secondary hypertension: an age-based approach. Am Fam Phys. 2010;82(12):1471-8.

20. Webb R, Mathur A, Chang R, et al. What is the best criterion for the interpretation of adrenal vein sample results in patients with primary hyperaldosteronism? Ann Surg Oncol. 2012;19:1881-6.

21. Weinberger MH, Fineberg NS. The diagnosis of primary aldosteronism and separation of two major subtypes. Arch Intern Med. 1993;153:2125-9.

22. Young WF, Stanson AW, Thompson GB, et al. Role for adrenal venous sampling in primary aldosteronism. Surgery. 2004;136:1227-35.

23. Young WF. Primary aldosteronism: renaissance of a syndrome. Clin Endocrinol (Oxf). 2007;66:607-18.

24. Young WF Jr. Primary aldosteronism: diagnosis. In: Mansoor GA (Ed). Secondary Hypertension: Clinical Presentation, Diagnosis, and Treatment. Totowa, NJ: Humana Press; 2004. pp. 119-37.

16

CHAPTER **Precocious Puberty in Boys**

Anjana Hulse

INTRODUCTION

Puberty is a distinct period of sexual maturation that occurs during adolescence which is a developmental stage between childhood and adulthood. The onset of true puberty is marked by the development of breast bud in girls and increase in testicular volume (≥4 mL) in boys. Precocious puberty is defined as the development of secondary sexual characteristics before the age of 8 years in girls and 9 years in boys. The prevalence of precocious puberty is about ten times higher in girls than in boys. Commonest cause of precocious puberty in girls is idiopathic central precocious puberty. In contrast, precocious puberty in boys is often because of organic reasons. Hence, it is extremely important to evaluate boys who present with precocious puberty.

CASE HISTORY

A 6-year-old boy was referred with a history of recent onset pubic and axillary hair. His mother had noticed hair growth under his arms and over the pubic area since 3 months. She also complained of body odor. There was no history of vomiting, seizures or failure to thrive.

This boy was born at term weighing 3,500 g by spontaneous vaginal delivery. Pregnancy was uneventful except for one episode of urinary tract infection in the mother. The parents were nonconsanguineous. At birth there was cord around the neck. He did not cry immediately at birth but did so after a brief resuscitation with bag and mask. He required feeding support during neonatal period.

During infancy, the baby was noted to have delayed motor development. He developed spasticity in all four limbs. He was evaluated and was diagnosed with "spastic quadriplegic cerebral palsy." MRI which was done at the age of 9 months was normal. Now at the age of 6 years he had spasticity in all four limbs and was confined to bed. He was tall for his age (height 125 cm >97th centile, weight 26 kg >97th centile). He had coarse, dark pubic hair at the base of penis and also a few strands of hair in the axillary region. Both testes were about 8 mL in size and development of his genitalia corresponded to Tanner stage 3. Cardiovascular, abdominal, and respiratory examination was normal. He could just vocalize and understand a few simple commands but could not speak. Fundoscopy was normal.

Based on the above findings this patient was diagnosed to have precocious puberty. It is known that the children with cerebral palsy as well as other neurological disorders are at increased risk of developing early puberty. The diagnosis of precocious puberty in this boy was confirmed by further evaluation.

DISCUSSION

Precocious puberty is defined as development of secondary sexual characters before the age of 9 years in boys (before 8 years in girls). Precocious puberty may be gonadotropin dependent or gonadotropin independent. Precocious puberty is far more common in girls than in boys.

Isosexual and Heterosexual Precocious Puberty

Pubertal development of the same sex (e.g., feminization in a girl) is termed "isosexual precocious puberty." Pubertal development of the opposite sex is termed "heterosexual precocious puberty."

Clinical Features of Precocious Puberty in Boys

The first sign of onset of puberty in boys is an increase in testicular volume. Testicular volume can be measured accurately using a Prader orchidometer (**Fig. 1**). Testicular volume of ≥4 mL is considered as pubertal. In about

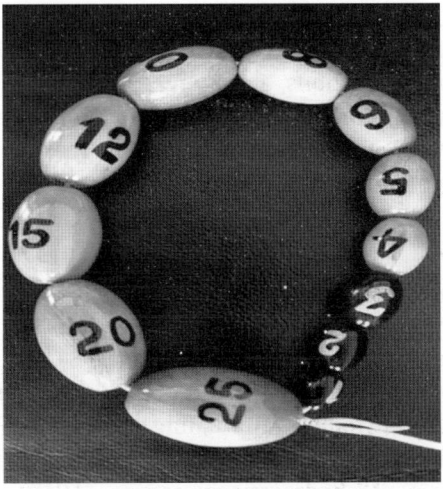

FIG. 1: Prader orchidometer. (***For color version, see plate 6***)

TABLE 1: Tanner staging of puberty in boys.

Stage	Genitalia	Pubic hair
1	Testes <4 mL, genitalia-prepubertal	Prepubertal
2	Testes >4 mL; scrotal skin reddens and changes in texture	Lightly pigmented, long hair at the base of penis
3	Further growth of testes 6–8 mL, lengthening of penis, further growth of scrotum	Darker and coarser hair over pubic symphysis
4	Testes 8–12 mL, further growth of penis in length and breadth, scrotal pigmentation	Adult pubic hair but confined to suprapubic area
5	Genitalia adult in size and shape, testes 15–25 mL	Adult hair may extend to thighs and lower abdomen

TABLE 2: Investigations for precocious puberty in boys.

Laboratory tests	Serum levels of LH, FSH, testosterone, TSH and free T4, Prolactin, DHEAS, 17OHP, beta HCG, AFP (as indicated)
	When indicated, provocation test using GnRH or GnRHa
Radiograph	AP view of the left hand and wrist to estimate skeletal age
Imaging	• Neuroimaging for all boys with gonadotropin dependent precocious puberty • Adrenal imaging, if indicated
Sonography	Ultrasound scan of testes when indicated

(17 OHP: 17 hydroxyprogesterone; AFP: alpha fetoprotein; DHEAS: dihydroepiandrostenedione sulfate; Free T4: free thyroxine; FSH: follicle-stimulating hormone; HCG: human chorionic gonadotropin; LH: luteinizing hormone; TSH: thyroid stimulating hormone; GnRH: gonadotropin-releasing hormone; GnRHa: gonadotropin-releasing hormone agonist; AP: anteroposterior)

20% of children, pubic hair growth may be the first sign of puberty. As the puberty progresses there will be gradual increase in testicular volume, increase in penile growth, and hair growth over the pubic and axillary area. **Table 1** describes Tanner staging of male puberty. Other androgen effects such as increase in muscle bulk and strength, acne, deepening of the voice, and eventually facial hair growth are seen in boys. Behavioral changes (aggression), frequent erections, and increased libido are expected to occur during puberty. Puberty in boys is associated with increase in growth velocity with peak height velocity of about 8–12 cm per year which occurs usually during Tanner stage 4 and 5.

Investigations

The clinical features listed in this case prompt us to suspect precocious puberty. When precocious puberty is suspected in boys, it warrants certain investigations in boys (**Table 2**).

This patient had his basal serum luteinizing hormone (S. LH) (0.2 mIU/mL) and serum follicle-stimulating hormone (S. FSH) (2.3 mIU/mL) levels checked. His testosterone level was 72.3 ng/dL. He was biochemically euthyroid. Prolactin, 17-hydroxyprogesterone (OHP), dihydroepiandrostenedione sulfate (DHEAS), and tumor markers were normal. The skeletal age was advanced by 4 years (skeletal age 10 years at a chronological age of 6 years). Since his basal gonadotropins were less than the pubertal level, a provocation test using injection Leuprorelin 1 mg was done which showed a pubertal response (peak S.LH 8.3 mIU/mL, S.FSH 5.7 mIU/mL). These findings confirm central precocious puberty (CPP). In view of his young age, an MRI of the pituitary was done. MRI showed normal pituitary and diffuse cerebral atrophy. Therefore, this patient who was a known case of cerebral palsy was diagnosed with idiopathic CPP.

Gonadotropin-releasing Hormone Agonist Stimulation Test

Historically, provocative testing to diagnose precocious puberty was done using gonadotropin releasing hormone (GnRH). Currently, because of nonavailability of GnRH, analogs are being used for provocative tests to confirm puberty. GnRH analog testing also has the advantage of being performed on an outpatient basis with fewer sampling, when compared to the conventional GnRH stimulation test. Commonly used Gonadotropin-releasing Hormone Agonist (GnRHa) is leuprolide. There are various protocols but commonly used protocol involves using leuprolide 10–20 μg/kg (maximum 1 mg) as subcutaneous injection. Samples are taken for S.LH and S.FSH before (baseline) and 2–4 hours after leuprolide injection and for testosterone levels at 24 hours after leuprolide injection.

Other agents used for provocative tests include subcutaneous Triptorelin acetate (0.1 mg/m^2, to a maximum of 0.1 mg) with blood sampling at 0, 3 and 24 hours for LH, FSH, and for testosterone at 24 hours.

Generally, peak S.LH level of >5 mIU/mL and LH >FSH and serum testosterone levels >25 ng/dL is considered as pubertal response. However, GnRHa stimulation test results should be interpreted in the clinical context and on the background of radiological and laboratory tests performed to diagnose puberty.

Disorders Causing Precocious Puberty in Boys

Precocious puberty in boys could be gonadotropin dependent or CPP due to disorders of pituitary or hypothalamus or gonadotropin independent or peripheral precocious puberty due to disorders of adrenal glands or gonads. Sometimes, puberty may be a combination of gonadotropin dependent and gonadotropin independent precocious puberty. This occurs usually in chronic conditions such as congenital adrenal hyperplasia (CAH). This is thought to be because of triggering of hypothalamic–pituitary–adrenal (HPA) due to peripheral sexual precocity. Precocious puberty in boys always warrants evaluation as it is often pathological. Idiopathic CPP is common in girls. Various etiologies of precocious puberty in boys with their specific features are listed here in **Table 3**.

TABLE 3: Etiology of precocious puberty in boys.

Etiology	Specific features
Gonadotropin dependent	
Idiopathic	This is a diagnosis of exclusion. In contrast to girls, idiopathic central precocious in boys accounts for only 20% of cases of precocious puberty. Idiopathic CPP in boys results from early activation of normal HPA. Tempo of puberty may vary but usually puberty is complete by 2–4 years. GnRHa stimulation shows predominant LH response and neuroimaging is normal. In addition to psychological disturbances, short stature resulting from early epiphyseal fusion is the main concern
Hypothalamic hamartoma	These account for about 20% of cases of precocious puberty. Hamartomas are heterotopic isodense neuronal tissue commonly situated in the region of tuber cinereum sometimes may develop into pedunculated mass from the floor of third ventricle. Though the exact mechanism of precocious puberty in hamartoma is unknown it is believed that the hamartomas either produce GnRH or they interfere with the normal hypothalamic gonadostat. Clinical features are similar to idiopathic CPP though some cases may present with gelastic seizures. Signs of raised intracranial pressure, neurological deficits or visual disturbances are very rare. Management involves serial monitoring with neuroimaging and treatment of precocious puberty with GnRHa
CNS tumors	Pineal gland tumors may account for about 50% of cerebral causes of precocious puberty. These tumors may just present with precocious puberty or with the signs of raised intracranial pressure, other pituitary hormone deficiencies, neurological deficits or visual disturbances. A skull radiograph may show calcification of pineal gland. Other CNS tumors such as glioma, dysgerminoma, teratoma, craniopharyngioma, and prolactinoma can cause precocious puberty in boys. When CNS etiology is suspected, it is extremely important to take a careful history, carry out neurological and ophthalmological examination and MRI of the brain. Appropriate treatment of the tumor is essential. Puberty may be rapidly progressing in case of CNS tumors
CNS trauma, radiation	Head injury, radiation for head and neck tumor can also cause precocious puberty probably by interfering with the restrain on HPA
CNS malformations	CNS malformations such as septo-optic dysplasia, arachnoid cysts, hydrocephalus, and meningomyelocele can cause CPP. Clinical symptoms in these conditions are similar to that of idiopathic CPP
Primary hypothyroidism	Boys with untreated primary hypothyroidism may develop pseudo precocious puberty with penile and testicular enlargement. They are short and may have other features of hypothyroidism. This is the only cause of precocious puberty where skeletal age is delayed in contrast to other causes of precocious puberty. It is known that TSH has some activity at the FSH receptor, and high levels may stimulate sex steroid production. There may be pituitary hyperplasia (**Fig. 2**). Treatment is with levothyroxine after biochemical confirmation of primary hypothyroidism

Continued

Continued

Etiology	Specific features
Gonadotropin independent	
Adrenal tumors	Adrenal tumors account for about 22% of cases of precocious puberty in boys out of which majority is due to congenital adrenal hyperplasia. Secondary sexual characters with small testis should prompt the clinician to look for adrenal pathology. Adrenal carcinoma may present with clinical features of glucocorticoid excess
Testicular tumors	Testicular tumors account for about 5% of cases of precocious puberty in boys. Asymmetrical testicles or unilateral testicular enlargement goes strongly in favor of testicular tumors. Leydig cell tumors commonly cause precocious puberty followed by seminoma (which often causes gynecomastia). There is autonomous production of androgens and gonadotropin levels may be low
McCune-Albright syndrome	Less common in boys in comparison to girls. Precocity is due to autonomous production of testosterone from testes. Other clinical features such as bone cysts and Café au lait spots aid the diagnosis of this condition
Familial male precocious puberty	Familial male precocious puberty, also known as testotoxicosis results from LH receptor mutation. Boys start with early onset of secondary sexual characters with rapid progression leading to early epiphyseal fusion resulting in short stature. Basal LH and testosterone levels are high

(CPP: central precocious puberty; LH: luteinizing hormone; FSH: follicle-stimulating hormone CNS: central nervous system: HPA: hypothalamic– pituitary–adrenal)

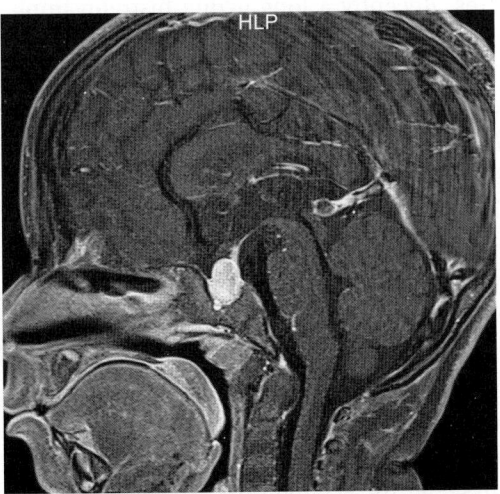

FIG. 2: Pituitary hyperplasia in a child with precocious puberty secondary to untreated primary hypothyroidism.

Treatment Options

This patient has gonadotropin-dependent precocious puberty. Gonadotropin-dependent precocious puberty warrants treatment with GnRH agonists. This boy was started on treatment with injection leuprolide acetate depot 11.25 mg to be given once in 3 months. In the past 2 years, there has been no progression of puberty following this treatment.

As seen in girls, precocious puberty in boys too, when untreated, can cause psychosocial problems and short stature. Excessive sex hormone production can cause early fusion of epiphysis leading to short adult height. Mismatch between psychosocial and physical growth may lead to withdrawn or aggressive behavior and early sexuality. Several treatment regimen using various GnRH agonists are used. GnRHa, downregulates gonadotropin receptors by constant stimulation. This downregulatory effect leads to inhibition of gonadotropin release by pituitary resulting in pubertal arrest, attenuation of skeletal advancement and a progressive increase in predicted adult height. Maximum benefit on height is achieved when treatment is started before 6 years of age at an early stage of puberty.

The most widely used GnRHa agents are leuprolide acetate (3.75–22.5 mg) intramuscular injection at a dose of 0.2–0.3 mg/kg every 4 weekly. Subcutaneous preparations (to be given every day) are used in some centers. Recently, depot preparations are being used commonly and found to be as effective as monthly preparations. Using depot preparations would obviate the need for monthly visits to the hospitals thereby improving the compliance. Various depot preparations are available including leuprolide depot (7.5 mg, 11.25 mg, and 22.5 mg), triptorelin pamoate and triptorelin acetate. An intranasal preparation of nafarelin acetate also is available in some countries. Recently a long-acting histrelin implant is being used increasingly in girls. It is inserted subcutaneously in an outpatient setting. The 50 mg implant provides continuous release of the potent GnRHa histrelin for over a year. Effective suppression of the hypothalamic-pituitary-gonadal (HPG) axis occurs within 1 month of its placement.

Use of depot preparations may sometimes be associated with sterile abscesses and pain at injection site. Anaphylaxis is a rare complication.

Monitoring Gonadotropin-releasing Hormone Agonist Therapy

Effectiveness and dosing adequacy of GnRHa is assessed based on clinical examination, hormonal assays and skeletal age. The patient is evaluated once in 4–6 months. Non progression of clinical signs and skeletal age on radiograph go in favor of effective dosing of GnRHa. In addition, S.LH levels measured 2 hours after the second dose of GnRHa depot injection helps to confirm suppression HPG axis.

What is the Rationale behind Adding Growth Hormone with Gonadotropin-releasing Hormone Agonist for Some Children with Precocious Puberty?

For some children with precocious puberty with advanced skeletal age, treatment with GnRHa may not be adequate to improve their final height.

For these children growth hormone (GH) therapy together with GnRHa is sometimes considered. As a consequence of gonadotropin or sex hormone suppression' there may be a dip in GH and insulin like growth factor 1 (IGF-1) production. This is the rationale behind combined therapy which is aimed at improving height gain.

Treatment of Gonadotropin Independent Precocious Puberty

Treatment of gonadotropin independent precocious puberty depends on the cause of puberty. Testicular or adrenal tumors need surgical excision. If there is metastasis, radiotherapy or chemotherapy may be needed depending on the type of tumor.

In cases of precocious puberty in a patient with CAH, appropriate gluco-corticoid replacement (and mineralocorticoid if needed) helps prevent progression of puberty. Careful monitoring and adjustment of the gluco-corticoid doses is required to achieve the maximum benefit. Precocious puberty associated with hypothyroidism is treated with thyroxine.

In familial male precocious puberty, ketoconazole has been tried. It is an antifungal agent which interferes with adrenal and gonadal 17,20 desmolase activity and to a lesser extent with 17 alpha hydroxylase and 11 beta hydroxylase activity. Other agents which have been used include cyproterone acetate, anastrozole, spironolactone, testolactone and bicalutamide. But these agents have shown minimal efficacy in attaining normal adult height. In recent studies, a combination of bicalutamide and anastrozole has been shown to be effective in treating familial male precocious puberty. Bicalutamide is a highly selective antiandrogen and anastrozole is a potent aromatase inhibitor.

What are the Problems a Child may Face Because of Precocious Puberty?

Just like girls, boys with precocious puberty too may have psychological and emotional problems as they look different compared to their peer group because of early onset of secondary sexual characters. This may result in these boys being the victims of bullying and teasing. The children may also show withdrawn or aggressive behavior. Parents or teachers may expect these children to perform better in terms of social interaction as well as physical activity as these children are bigger than their peer group. Since their psychosocial development is not advanced like their physical development, these children may not be able to cope with the higher expectations from their parents or teachers. These children need reassurance from their parents and teachers explaining that their body changes are normal but it is just that it has happened earlier for them.

Are Children with Neurodevelopmental Problems at Increased Risk of Precocious Puberty?

The children with a neurodevelopmental problem are at increased risk of developing signs of early puberty compared to the children without neurodevelopmental disability. A child with a neurodevelopmental disability is 20 times more likely to develop early puberty when compared to normal children. This calls for regular monitoring of these children to detect the signs of early puberty at the earliest. In children with cerebral palsy, it is known that puberty begins early but it is completed later than the general population.

Mention One Condition Causing Precocious Puberty Where Skeletal Age is Delayed

Untreated hypothyroidism can cause precocious puberty. Generally in precocious puberty skeletal age is advanced, but in precocious puberty resulting from hypothyroidism, skeletal age is delayed.

CONCLUSION

Prompt recognition and evaluation of boys with precocious puberty is necessary not only to avoid undesirable psychological and physical consequences, but also to diagnose underlying pathology if there is any.

SUGGESTED READINGS

1. Almeida MQ, Brito VN, Lins TS, et al. Long-term treatment of familial male-limited precocious puberty (testotoxicosis) with cyproterone acetate or ketoconazole. Clin Endocrinol (Oxf). 2008;69(1):93-8.
2. Freire AV, Escobar ME, Gryngarten MG, et al. High diagnostic accuracy of subcutaneous Triptorelin test compared with GnRH test for diagnosing central precocious puberty in girls. Clin Endocrinol (Oxf). 2013;78(3):398-404.
3. Ibanez L, Potau N, Zampolli M, et al. Use of leuprolide acetate response patterns in the early diagnosis of pubertal disorders: comparison with the gonadotropin-releasing hormone test. J Clin Endocrinol Metab. 1994;78(1):30-5.
4. Lifshitz F. Pediatric Endocrinology, 1st edition. Hoboken: Taylor and Francis; 2013.
5. Mitre N, Lteif A. Treatment of familial male-limited precocious puberty (testotoxicosis) with anastrozole and bicalutamide in a boy with a novel mutation in the luteinizing hormone receptor. J Pediatr Endocrinol Metab. 2009;22(12):1163-7.
6. Poomthavorn P, Khlairit P, Mahachoklertwattana P. Subcutaneous gonadotropin-releasing hormone agonist (triptorelin) test for diagnosing precocious puberty. Horm Res. 2009;72(2):114-9.
7. Prasad HK, Khadilkar VV, Jahagirdar R, et al. Evaluation of GnRH analogue testing in diagnosis and management of children with pubertal disorders. Indian J Endocr Metab. 2012;16(3):400-5.
8. Siddiqi SU,Van Dyke DC, Donohoue P, et al. Premature sexual development in individuals with neurodevelopmental disabilities. Dev Med Child Neurol. 1999;41(6):392-5.
9. Sperling M. Pediatric Endocrinology, 3rd edition. Amsterdam: Elsevier; 2008.
10. Worley G, Houlihan CM, Herman-Giddens ME, et al. Secondary sexual characteristics in children with cerebral palsy and moderate to severe motor impairment: a cross-sectional survey. Paediatrics. 2002;110(5):897-902.

17

CHAPTER

Approach to a Case of Gynecomastia

Sweety Agarwal, Priyanka Choudhry, Mohd Ashraf Ganie

INTRODUCTION

Gynecomastia is defined as the enlargement of the glandular tissue of the male breast. It is a common condition, seen in up to two-thirds of all adult men, and histologically in half of all men at autopsy. Most cases are benign, but it can be the manifestation of an underlying systemic disease.

Estrogen and growth hormone and insulin-like growth factor-1 (IGF-1) are required for the growth of a male breast. A balance exists between estrogens and androgens in males. Any disease state or medication that increases circulating estrogens or decreases circulating androgens can increase the estrogen to androgen ratio, causing gynecomastia. The estrogen effect on the breast can be due to either circulating estradiol levels or locally produced estrogen. Estrogens are locally produced by aromatization of androgens by aromatase P50 enzyme. An excess of this enzyme's substrate or an increase in enzyme activity can, thus, lead to gynecomastia.

There are many causes of gynecomastia and diagnosis is usually made after proper physical examination and investigations. Drug-induced gynecomastia is common and it is imperative to take a detailed drug history in any patient who presents with symptoms of breast enlargement. We present a case of spironolactone-induced gynecomastia in whom we ruled out other causes and symptoms improved after drug withdrawal.

CASE REPORT

Mr SS, a 48-year-old male, known hypertensive for 10 years duration, was on amlodipine 10 mg once daily, with which his blood pressure was well controlled. He was evaluated 2 years back for recurrent quadriparesis episodes (six to seven such episodes), without any sensory loss, bladder and bowel involvement, or sensorium alteration. He had severe hypokalemia. A diagnosis of hypokalemic periodic paralysis was made and the patient started on oral potassium replacement, after which there was no recurrence. Further, evaluation for the cause of hypokalemia revealed a raised aldosterone-to-renin ratio (74:4) with an absolute aldosterone concentration of 49.1 ng/dL. A contrast-enhanced CT scan of the abdomen was done and revealed a 1.1 × 1 cm round well-defined lesion of 24.5 Hounsfield units in the lateral limb of the left adrenal gland with 92.2% washout, suggestive of an adenoma. A diagnosis of primary aldosteronism was made and he was advised surgery, which the patient declined. Following this, he was started on spironolactone 100 mg once a day as medical management. Up to 2 months after starting spironolactone, the patient noticed a painful enlargement of both breasts. There was no associated discharge. He also noticed erectile dysfunction. There was no history of jaundice, facial/periorbital puffiness, or other hepatic or renal disease signs. There was no history of testicular trauma or infection. Breast enlargement was progressive and he stopped the drug 6 weeks before presentation to us. After discontinuation of the drug, the pain has subsided and sexual dysfunction has improved. He had evidence of glandular tissue of 4 cm palpable on each side, which was nontender on presentation. There was no hepatomegaly, pedal edema, or jaundice. Genital examination revealed normal bilateral testes with a volume of 20 mL on either side and no palpable mass.

Investigations were done to rule out other causes of gynecomastia. Liver function tests were normal with a serum glutamic oxaloacetic transaminase (SGOT) of 27 IU/L and serum glutamic pyruvic transaminase (SGPT) of 58 IU/L. Blood urea was 26 mg/dL and serum creatinine value of 0.4 mg/dL, indicating normal renal function. The thyroid function test was within normal limits [thyroxine (T4): 8.81 µg/dL and thyroid-stimulating hormone (TSH): 3.35 µIU/mL]. Serum testosterone value was 299 ng/dL (normal: 270–1,070 ng/dL) and prolactin was 11.96 ng/mL (normal: <20 ng/mL). The systemic examination and investigations were within normal limits.

The patient had already reported improvement in symptoms after stopping spironolactone. A diagnosis of drug-induced gynecomastia was made.

The patient is currently being evaluated for hyperaldosteronism and definitive treatment is planned for it.

DISCUSSION

Drugs cause an estimated 10–25% of gynecomastia cases and multiple medications have been implicated. Drugs with good evidence for association with gynecomastia are spironolactone, cimetidine, ketoconazole, growth hormone, gonadotropins, and antiandrogens such as 5-alpha-reductase inhibitors. Other drugs with an acceptable quality of evidence for association with gynecomastia are risperidone, calcium channel blockers, omeprazole, alkylating agents, anabolic steroids, alcohol, and opioids.

After initiation of spironolactone, gynecomastia can develop as early as after 1 month. In a trial of 30 men given spironolactone 100 mg, 200 mg, and placebo, gynecomastia developed in 3 out of 10 men in the 100 mg/day group, 5 out of 8 men in the 200 mg/day group, and none in the 12 men receiving placebo. Spironolactone binds to the androgen receptors and acts as an antiandrogen. It also increases testosterone's metabolic clearance, displaces estrogen from sex hormone-binding globulin (SHBG), and increases testosterone's peripheral conversion to estrogen.

Drug-induced gynecomastia is widespread. A thorough drug history may avoid unnecessary investigations in a particular case. Withdrawal of the offending drug, if possible, is the appropriate treatment for such cases.

APPROACH TO GYNECOMASTIA

There are no well-defined clinical thresholds to describe gynecomastia. Various authors have used varying definitions ranging from 0.5 to 3 cm of palpable glandular tissue. Gynecomastia is secondary to an imbalance between free estrogen and free androgen actions in the breast tissue. It occurs when there is an absolute or relative deficiency of androgens, deficient androgen action, or estrogen increase. The various causes of gynecomastia are listed in **Box 1**.

BOX 1 | **Etiology of gynecomastia.**

- *Absolute estrogen excess*:
  - Exogenous estrogens
  - *Endogenous production from*:
    - Testis—Leydig cell tumors, Sertoli cell tumors, and human chorionic gonadotropin (HCG)-secreting tumors
    - Adrenal—feminizing adrenocortical tumors
  - Increased aromatization—drugs, aromatase excess syndrome, aging, obesity, and hyperthyroidism
- *Absolute androgen deficiency*:
  - *Primary hypogonadism*:
    - Klinefelter syndrome
    - Testicular trauma
    - Chemotherapeutics
    - Infection
    - Radiation
  - *Secondary hypogonadism*:
    - Pituitary disease
    - Hypothalamic disease
- *Altered androgen-to-estrogen ratio*:
  - Puberty
  - Aging
  - Refeeding gynecomastia
  - Renal failure and dialysis
  - Hepatic cirrhosis
  - Hyperthyroidism
- *Decreased androgen action*:
  - Drugs—spironolactone, bicalutamide, and cimetidine
  - Androgen receptor defects

Hypogonadism, whether primary as in Klinefelter syndrome, testicular injury due to drugs, radiation, chemotherapy, or secondary due to pituitary or hypothalamic causes, is the leading cause of gynecomastia. The mechanism is that the decrease in testosterone causes an increased estrogen/testosterone ratio. Klinefelter syndrome has the clinical features of small firm testes and a eunuchoid habitus.

Anabolic steroids can cause functional hypogonadism by inhibiting gonadotropin-releasing hormone, follicle-stimulating hormone (FSH), and luteinizing hormone (LH). Functional hypogonadism leads to a decrease in testicular volume and endogenous production of testosterone. Many anabolic steroids can be aromatized, leading to increased estrogen levels and imbalanced androgen-to-estrogen ratio.

The androgen resistance syndromes partial and complete due to testicular feminization have gynecomastia. This is because of the decreased androgen responsiveness at the breast level and increases estrogen levels due to elevated androgen precursors' aromatization to estradiol.

Physiological gynecomastia can occur in three phases of life. Shortly after birth, the high maternal estradiol and progesterone levels are responsible; this can last several weeks and produce mild breast discharge. Pubertal gynecomastia may be caused by decreased androgen production or increased aromatization of circulating androgens, increasing the androgen-to-estrogen ratio. It is common and up to 60% of boys can have gynecomastia by age of 14 years. Pubertal gynecomastia can be unilateral or bilateral and usually resolves within 3 years of onset. The third phase in which physiological gynecomastia occurs is old age >60 years. In old age, mild hypogonadism and increased peripheral aromatase activity secondary to increased total body fat cause gynecomastia.

PATHOLOGICAL GYNECOMASTIA

Tumors

Testicular tumors can cause increased blood estrogen levels through multiple mechanisms: Estrogen overproduction, androgen overproduction with aromatization in the periphery to estrogens, and ectopic secretion of gonadotropins, which stimulate normal Leydig cells.

Estrogen-producing tumors are Leydig cell tumors, Sertoli cell tumors, granulosa cell tumors, and adrenal tumors.

Leydig Cell Tumors

Leydig cell tumors constitute 1–3% of testicular tumors. Their usual age of presentation is between ages 20 and 60 years, but 25% can present prepubertally. The clinical presentation in prepubertal cases is isosexual precocity, rapid somatic growth, and increased bone age with increased serum testosterone. They present with elevated estrogen levels with a testicular mass on ultrasound of scrotum and gynecomastia in adults. They are usually benign, but rarely malignant with metastasis to the lungs, liver, and retroperitoneal lymph nodes.

Sertoli Cell Tumors

- Gynecomastia occurs in one-third of Sertoli cell tumors due to increased estrogen production. They occur at all ages and 10% can be malignant.
- Granulosa cell tumors are very rare; they overproduce estrogen and gynecomastia occurs in half of them.

Germ Cell Tumors

It is the most common cancer in males 15–35 years of age.

- They are divided into seminomatous and nonseminomatous subtypes and include embryonal carcinoma, yolk cell carcinoma, choriocarcinomas, and teratomas.
- Increased HCG levels and alpha-fetoprotein are reliable markers in some tumors.
- The increased HCG levels, analogous to LH levels, stimulate the Leydig cells to secrete extratesticular estrogens, which cause gynecomastia.

NONTUMOR CAUSES OF GYNECOMASTIA

Increased Aromatase Activity

Tumors, drugs, obesity, and hyperthyroidism can cause gynecomastia by excessive aromatization of androgens to estrogens. New genetic causes of gynecomastia have been found. A familial form of gynecomastia has been discovered in which there is elevation of extragonadal aromatase activity. A novel gain of function mutation in chromosome 15 causes gynecomastia by forming cryptic promoters that lead to overexpression of aromatase.

DIAGNOSTIC EVALUATION OF GYNECOMASTIA

The first step is a thorough history of the duration of gynecomastia, breast pain, and nipple discharge. A history of renal and liver disease is necessary, as they are important causes of gynecomastia. A detailed sexual history about libido, erectile dysfunction, and regression of secondary sexual characteristics should be taken, as these symptoms point toward hypogonadism as the cause. Abnormal weight points to a diagnosis of lipomastia or pseudogynecomastia. Symptoms of hyperthyroidism are to be enquired. Finally, detailed drug history, including recreational drug use and history of dietary or occupational exposure to estrogen, is to be taken to rule out drug-induced gynecomastia.

Physical examination is done to differentiate true gynecomastia from pseudogynecomastia. Pseudogynecomastia is characterized by an increase in subareolar fat alone in the absence of glandular enlargement. Comparing the subareolar tissue with adjacent subcutaneous fat in the anterior axillary fold is done for this. A firm mound of tissue is found around the areola in true gynecomastia. The gynecomastia can be unilateral or bilateral and symmetric or asymmetric. The small size of the testes and soft consistency, small penile size, decreased pubic hair, and absence of facial and axillary hair are important signs to look at as they indicate hypogonadism. Hepatosplenomegaly, ascites, and pedal edema point to liver disease. The patient is examined for tremors, goiter, and eye signs of thyrotoxicosis.

Investigations are done to find the cause. Liver and renal functions are done. Free triiodothyronine (FT3), free thyroxine (FT4), TSH, LH, FSH, testosterone, and prolactin in three pooled samples are taken. Serum beta-HCG and X-ray chest posteroanterior (PA) are done. These investigations are done in all patients to rule out liver and renal dysfunction, hypogonadism, and HCG-secreting germ cell tumors. The scrotum's ultrasound is done, if a testicular tumor is suspected, and a CT or MRI of the abdomen is done, if an adrenal tumor is suspected. Mammography and ultrasound of breasts are indicated only, if breast carcinoma is suspected.

The mechanism of gynecomastia in liver and renal dysfunction is altered androgen-to-estradiol ratio. In thyrotoxicosis, there are increased levels of SHBG and aromatization of androgen to estrogen. Hypogonadism causes decreased testosterone and in germ cell tumors secreting estrogen, the increased estrogen alters the androgen-to-estradiol ratio. Hyper-prolactinemia leads to hypogonadism, thus indirectly decreasing the testosterone/estradiol ratio.

MANAGEMENT OF GYNECOMASTIA

No treatment is required for asymptomatic pubertal gynecomastia. Prolonged asymptomatic gynecomastia requires no treatment, except for cosmetic reasons.

Weight loss is the treatment for pseudogynecomastia or lipomastia, but it does not work, then plastic surgery is done.

If gynecomastia is progressive or associated with breast pain, evaluation should be done to find the cause. If a reversible cause is found, then the cause is treated. Every symptomatic patient with gynecomastia should be subjected to medical therapy or surgical therapy.

Medical Therapy

Medical therapy is effective, if the disease onset is <2 years because, after 2 years, fibrosis of the stroma sets in. Tamoxifen is the first line of treatment. The dose is 10–20 mg daily 3–9 months and has shown the efficacy of up to 90% for gynecomastia resolution. A second course may be given, if gynecomastia recurs. Tamoxifen has been used as a prophylaxis against gynecomastia in patients with prostate carcinoma treated with antiandrogens. Raloxifene was found useful in 92% of cases and clomiphene citrate was found useful in 42% of cases. Anastrozole, an aromatase inhibitor, has also been used, but it is not as effective as antiestrogens. In men with hypogonadism, testosterone therapy is used. Testosterone, sometimes, worsens gynecomastia due to aromatization to estrogens. Dihydrotestosterone, which is a nonaromatizable androgen, has been used topically to treat gynecomastia.

Surgical Therapy

The indications for surgery are painful gynecomastia, to relieve psychological stress, for cosmetic reasons, in suspected malignancy, in long-standing gynecomastia >12 months duration, and patients not responsive to medical therapy.

The surgical procedure used most often is a subcutaneous reduction mammoplasty, in which direct resection of glandular tissue is done using a periareolar or subareolar approach with liposuction.

If the breast enlargement is purely due to fat tissue without glandular hyperplasia, then liposuction alone gives satisfactory results.

CONCLUSION

Gynecomastia is a common physical finding, but it may be the sign of an underlying disease. Hence, adequate evaluation is needed to identify the etiology and guide appropriate therapy. Pseudogynecomastia has to be differentiated from true gynecomastia. Physiological causes of gynecomastia such as infancy, adolescence, and old age need no treatment.

Gynecomastia, which is progressive or painful, has to be treated. Medical therapy works only, if the duration of gynecomastia is <2 years.

When medical option fails, the surgical option of reduction mammoplasty is used.

SUGGESTED READINGS

1. Braunstein GD. Clinical practice. Gynecomastia. N Engl J Med. 2007;357:1229-37.
2. Carlson HE. Gynecomastia. N Engl J Med. 1980;303:795-9.
3. Cuhaci N, Polat SB, Evranos B, Ersoy R, Cakir B. Gynecomastia: Clinical evaluation and management. Indian J Endocrinol Metab. 2014;18:150-8.
4. Deepinder F, Braunstein GD. Drug-induced gynecomastia: an evidence-based review. Expert Opin Drug Saf. 2012;11:779-95.
5. Dobs A, Darkes MJM. Incidence and management of gynecomastia in men treated for prostate cancer. J Urol. 2005;174:1737-42.
6. Georgiadis E, Papandreou L, Evangelopoulou C, Aliferis C, Lymberis C, Panitsa C, et al. Incidence of gynecomastia in 954 young males and its relationship to somatometric parameters. Ann Hum Biol. 1994;21:579-87.
7. Huffman DH, Kampmann JP, Hignite CE, Azarnoff DL. Gynecomastia induced in normal males by spironolactone. Clin Pharmacol Ther. 1978;24:465-73.
8. Nuttall FQ. Gynecomastia as a physical finding in normal men. J Clin Endocrinol Metab. 1979;48:338-40.
9. Williams MJ. Gynecomastia. Its incidence, recognition and host characterization in 447 autopsy cases. Am J Med. 1963;34:103-12.

18
CHAPTER Menopause

Srinivasa P Munigoti, Archana Ramesh

INTRODUCTION

Menopause in women is a result of cessation of ovulation due to loss of ovarian follicles. Reduced estrogen levels that follow this process leads to clinical symptoms such as irregular cycles followed by complete cessation of menstrual flow, vasomotor symptoms and accelerated bone loss increasing the risk of osteoporosis and fractures of the bone. This chapter explores these issues related to menopause, starting with clinical presentation and possible therapeutic options based on the latest evidence.

CASE HISTORY

A 49-year-old female presents with history of "hot flushes" and "night sweats". Her last menstrual period was a year ago. She complains of dryness of vagina and severe pain on sexual intercourse. She also complains of frequent micturition and dysuria. She also has hypertension for which she is on medication and reports a strong family history of early heart disease and diabetes. She has been advised by her family doctor to undergo bone mineral density (BMD) spine (lumbar vertebrae) which showed "T-score of -2.2". She is keen to explore therapeutic options to improve her health that includes her symptoms, cardiovascular, and bone health

Going back to the clinical case, HRT should be the first treatment of choice for her vasomotor symptoms. If HRT is used, it may also in addition provide some protection against bone loss and she may not need to consider any alternatives for osteopenia till the time she remains on HRT. She may need vitamin D supplementation, if inadequate, and she should also be counseled about diet that meets her daily calcium need. Given no proven benefit of HRT in reducing her CVD risk, one should consider alternative treatment options that include regular exercise, balanced diet, statin therapy, and antihypertensive drugs toward reducing her cardiovascular risk.

DISCUSSION

Menopause

Menopause is defined as the cessation of menstruation which reflects absence of ovulation due to loss of ovarian follicles, and estrogen as a consequence. Average menopausal age worldwide is 51 years, whereas that of an Indian woman is 46.2 years, much less than their western counterparts.

Diagnosis of menopause remains clinical. It is made in women who have not had a period for at least 12 months whilst not using hormonal contraception. A singular and consistent rise in follicle-stimulating hormone (FSH) is often seen as an important hormonal biomarker of the menopausal transition. Such a rise in FSH is recognized to be more sustained over time in the early years after the last menstrual period. Hence, serial measurement of FSH can be a useful in a woman aged 40–45 years, presenting with a change in their menstrual cycle and/or vasomotor symptoms.

Ovarian failure leading to menopause, most frequently presents with vasomotor symptoms, mood disorders, urogenital atrophy and sexual dysfunction influencing women's quality of life and in longer term leading to increased risk of fragility fractures secondary to osteoporosis. These short- and long-term sequelae related to menopause are sometimes loosely referred to as "postmenopausal syndrome". Whereas, estrogen deficiency associated increased cardiovascular risk is well recognized, estrogen replacement as a treatment for the same has not been supported by several well-conducted clinical trials.

Vasomotor Symptoms

Vasomotor symptoms described as hot flushes and night sweats, affects about 70% of women and very significantly in about 20%, during menopause often bringing them into medical attention. These symptoms usually last for about 5 years but may continue for many more years in about 10% of women. Underlying pathophysiology of hot flushes remains poorly understood. According to one proposed theory, estrogen withdrawal leading to a decrease in endorphin and catecholestrogen levels and to an increased norepine-phrine and serotonin release is thought to cause peripheral vasodilatation and an altered "set point" in the thermoregulatory nucleus leading to hot flushes, and night sweats.

Low dose oral contraceptive pills (OCPs) may be the first therapeutic choice in perimenopausal women who are still menstruating. In menopausal women, conjugated estrogens, oral or as transdermal patches are proven to be effective. Hormone replacement therapy (HRT) is not only proven to be effective in relieving vasomotor symptoms but also is shown to be beneficial in improving mood and any associated depression.

Clonidine available as oral tablets given at doses of 0.1–0.2 mg/day is known to provide relief and is thought to act by reducing central nor-adrenergic tone. In some studies, paroxetine, a selective serotonin reuptake inhibitor (with a starting dose of 25 mg/day) has been shown to reduce both frequency and severity of vasomotor symptoms. Similarly, gabapentin (300–900 mg/day), venlafaxine (starting with 75 mg/day), and citalopram (starting with 10 mg/day) have also been tried and shown to be of varied success in providing relief from vasomotor symptoms.

A common practice though is vitamin E supplementation. About 120 women subjected to a randomized, cross-over, clinical trial received vitamin E (800 IU daily) or placebo for 4 weeks and vice-versa for another 4 weeks. On crossover analysis, vitamin E was associated with a reduction of hot flushes.

Weight loss with lifestyle modifications is actually found to reduce the severity and hence it should be recommended appropriately in all women.

Urogenital Atrophy

Owing to loss of integrity of urothelial lining of the lower urinary tract, symptoms such as dysuria, frequency, urgency with recurrent infections are presenting features in >50% of postmenopausal women. Similarly dryness, superficial dyspareunia and sometimes bleeding reflect changes in vaginal mucosa and secretions. Both systemic and local estrogens help in alleviation of these symptoms. Low-doses of estrogen cream (0.5 g) are found effective only when used 1–3 times weekly. Estrogen-releasing vaginal ring or estradiol vaginal tablet (25 µg) inserted twice weekly may be convenient and easier to use than estrogen cream. However, these women should be counseled about importance of seeking medical attention if they notice any bleeding whilst on therapy. Lubricants, a nonhormonal alternative for dyspareunia may be recommended in the presence of already existent urogenital atrophy where HRT may not be of any use.

Sexual Dysfunction

Prevalence of sexual dysfunction in perimenopausal age group is reported to be about 43%. However, careful evaluation of physical, psychological, lifestyle factors, and relationship variables for optimal therapy is essential as it is often complex and multifactorial. In a double-blind, crossover study involving surgically menopausal women, intramuscular testosterone given in supra physiological doses (female reference) resulted in significantly higher scores of sexual desire and arousal than did treatment with estradiol alone or placebo. In another study comparing methyltestosterone (1.25 mg/day) combined with esterified estrogens (0.625 mg/day), with estrogen alone, women treated with combination pill that included testosterone showed increased sexual desire and libido compared to those treated with estrogen alone. Whenever, androgenic combinations are used, it is important to counsel patients about potential side-effects like hirsutism, acne, deepening of voice, altered lipid profile, and liver function.

Osteoporosis

Accelerated bone loss following menopause due to increase in the rate of bone turnover results in osteoporosis. This is widely recognized to be the result of lack of estrogen. World Health Organization/International Osteoporosis Foundation (WHO/IOF) identifies osteoporosis as "a systemic skeletal disease characterized by low bone mass (measured as BMD) and microarchitectural deterioration of bone tissue with a consequent increase in bone fragility and susceptibility to fractures involving the wrist, spine, hip and pelvis" and defines osteoporosis based on value for BMD –2.5 SD or more assessed at the femoral neck below that of a young female adult mean (T-score ≤ –2.5 SD).

Estimates suggest that 20% women amongst 230 million Indians over the age of 50 years in 2015 are osteoporotic. Data on prevalence of osteoporosis among women in India is reported to be between 8% and 62% by numerous studies that included women of various age groups, conducted in small groups spread across the country.

Given that osteoporosis is a painless disease, prevention of fractures secondary to it causing pain, disability, and reduction in lifespan remains a prime motive for treatment. Analysis of published data from across the world shows that 50% of women with hip fracture never regain their functional independence and one-fifth of them die within 1 year of the fracture. Therefore, identifying women at the highest risk is a clinical priority. The risk of fragility fracture has been shown to increase by a factor of 2–3 for each 1-SD decrease in BMD measured at hip.

The "FRAX" scoring is well validated and widely accepted tool used across the world to identify patients with high risk of future fractures. The scores from the tool are designed to predict 10-year absolute risk for a fracture in an individual. It helps in risk stratification of fracture risk even in the absence of BMD and hence, it is a very useful tool in clinical practice. It should be borne in mind that heterogeneity in different populations spread across India and the prevalence of nutritional and other risk factors that may be unique to the Indian population are not considered in the calculation of FRAX scores.

Treatment

Lifestyle changes that include a diet rich in calcium (>800 mg/day) and exposure to sunlight or vitamin D supplementation to achieve a daily requirement of 1000 IU is a universal recommendation. In addition, regular weight-bearing and muscle-strengthening exercises are also advocated to maintain muscle strength, agility, and bone health.

Hormone replacement therapy (HRT) using either estrogen alone or in combination with progesterone has been shown to prevent osteoporotic fractures even in low-risk population. With an average follow-up of 5.2 years, HRT has been shown to increase lumbar spine BMD and femoral neck BMD, and consequently bringing down both hip and clinical vertebral fracture rates were shown to reduce significantly by 34% and all osteoporotic fractures by 24%. The dose and duration of HRT nevertheless, should be individualized, and a risk-benefit assessment should be carried out on a yearly basis. Indian guidelines also suggest mammogram to be carried out 1–3 yearly if the initial mammogram is normal on patients using HRT.

Data, from cumulative analysis of data gathered from routine clinical practice and opinions from various experts across the country regarding the use of HRT as a treatment in perimenopausal osteoporosis, has revealed that most clinicians would prefer HRT as a treatment option in early menopausal women with vasomotor symptoms as it serves dual purpose and most of them would shift their patients to bisphosphonates in due course of time keeping with the current understanding of advantages and disadvantages of HRT as discussed in the subsequent paragraphs.

Tibolone is a synthetic steroid with selective tissue estrogenic activity that also has progestogenic and androgenic properties. With its estrogenic effect on bone, it inhibits bone resorption by reducing osteoclastic activity. Tibolone at 2.5 mg/day has been proven to minimize bone loss and reduce the risk of vertebral and nonvertebral fracture in older osteoporotic women and is shown to be as effective as standard doses of conventional postmenopausal hormone therapy. In addition, tibolone is also proven to be effective in treating vasomotor symptoms and improves urogenital atrophy, making it a useful alternative to HRT.

Amongst nonhormonal treatments, bisphosphonates are recommended as first-line drugs for treating postmenopausal women, with proven efficacy in the prevention of vertebral and nonvertebral fractures, including hip fractures. Alendronate 70 mg weekly for up to 10 years is shown to produce a sustained increase in BMD with a significant reduction in spine fracture and a good safety profile. In a meta-analysis of 11 trials using alendronate therapy in postmenopausal women, the relative risk reduction of vertebral fractures in patients given a dose of 10 mg daily was 45% and nonvertebral fractures up to 16%. Improvements in bone density with alendronate increased with both dose and time.

Similarly, treatment with zoledronic acid (5 mg by intravenous infusion over at least 15 minute once yearly) has been shown to reduce the incidence of vertebral fracture by 70% over 3 years with significant reduction seen by 1 year. Rate of hip fracture is also reduced by 41% and any nonvertebral fracture by 25% over 3 years.

Teriparatide is an anabolic agent that works primarily by increasing bone formation rather than by decreasing resorption. In a trial involving women with low BMD and previous vertebral fractures, teriparatide (20 µg/day) used for 21 months, was associated with a lower risk of vertebral fractures by 65% and nonvertebral fractures by 35% when compared with placebo. Teriparatide available as an injectable at 20 µg/day dosage may be given subcutaneously on daily basis for 2 years, with or without concomitant use of bisphosphonates. After discontinuation of teriparatide, its benefits are quickly lost, if antiresorptive therapy is not started as a follow-up therapy.

Denosumab was the first biologic therapy approved to treat osteoporosis. It acts by inhibiting bone resorption via binding to the receptor activator of nuclear factor-κβ ligand (RANKL), effectively decreasing the differentiation of osteoclasts. Unlike bisphosphonates, it can be used in patients with compromised renal function. A study involving postmenopausal women with a BMD, T-score of < –2.5 but not < –4.0 at the lumbar spine (or) total hip showed that treatment with denosumab 60 mg given twice yearly via subcutaneous route resulted in a significantly lower risk of vertebral fractures by 68%, hip fractures by 40%, and nonvertebral fractures by 20% when compared to placebo.

Cardiovascular Disease

Heart and Estrogen/Progestin Replacement Study (HERS I and II)

Epidemiological studies in the 1970s identified cardiovascular disease (CVD) as the most important cause of mortality in both sexes, with an earlier prevalence in those with early menopause; thus, highlighting the protective role of estrogen. Heart and Estrogen/Progestin Replacement Study (HERS) were the first study designed to identify the prevention of recurrence of coronary heart disease (CHD) in a woman already suffering from it (secondary prevention). HERS involved 2,763 postmenopausal women with an average age of 67, who were treated with HRT for approximately 4 years. Results from this pivotal study showed us that women on conjugated equine estrogen (CEE) plus medroxyprogesterone acetate (MPA) did not show any cardiovascular benefit but instead had an increased incidence of venous thromboembolism (VTE) and gallbladder disease. On subanalysis of data from HERS I, a slight improvement in the CVD outcomes in patients with longer duration of therapy then led to extension of this study—HERS II. Results from this follow-up showed that lower rates of CHD events among women in the hormone group in the final years of HERS I did not persist during additional years of follow-up in HERS II. After 6.8 years of follow-up, hormone therapy did not reduce risk of cardiovascular events in women with CHD.

Women's Health Initiative Study

The Women's Health Initiative (WHI) study was launched in 1991, consisting of a set of clinical trials and an observational study, involving 161,808 postmenopausal women. This was the first randomized trial to address the effects of HRT on CHD incidence in predominantly healthy women with no prior history of CHD (primary prevention) unlike in HERS (secondary prevention) and this study also looked at the overall risks and benefits of HRT.

This trial included two studies, one was the estrogen-plus-progestin study of women with a uterus and the other being estrogen-alone study of women without a uterus. The combined arm of CEE + MPA had to be terminated prematurely in 2003 due to the detrimental effects noticed like breast cancer, stroke, VTE, and heart disease in spite of a decrease in fragile fractures, bowel cancers and diabetes. Estrogen only (CEE) arm of the trial, though, was continued. The study concluded that use of HRT did not offer any protection against increased CVD risk. Secondary subgroup analysis of the same study showed that CHD tended to be nonsignificantly reduced by HRT in younger women or women with <10 years since menopause. A small reduction in risk of total mortality was also noticed. Although not statistically significant, this conclusion from secondary analysis suggested that the effect of hormones on CHD may be modified by years since menopause, with the highest CVD risks in women who were 20 or more years since menopause (or aged ≥70 years).

The absence of excess absolute risk of CHD and the suggestion of reduced total mortality in younger women was reassuring and pointed toward a possibility that use of HRT may be a reasonable option for the short-term treatment of menopausal symptoms, but did not confirm or imply an absence of harm in their longer term use. Results from a number of similar smaller studies on the use of HRT in preventing CVD have confirmed no benefit.

Given this paucity of data to support use of HRT in mitigating the increased CVD risk, clinicians should focus on other preventive strategies such as appropriate treatment of hypercholesterolemia and any other coexistent illnesses such as type 2 diabetes mellitus (T2DM), hypertension, and obesity with lifestyle measures as well as medication as need be.

Hormone Replacement Therapy—Other Risks

Cancer

Breast

Women's Health Initiative study showed that use of combined HRT for 5 years increased the risk of breast cancer (1 extra case/1,000 women annually). On the contrary, collaborative analysis of data from 51 epidemiological studies involving 52,705 women with breast cancer and 108,411 women without breast cancer showed that "estrogen only" therapy actually lead to statistically significant decrease in breast cancer.

Ovary

Available data linking HRT and ovarian carcinoma is conflicting. Whilst WHI concluded that there was no change in the incidence, the Danish National Cancer registry revealed a small but significant increase in those using HRT for at least 8 years, either using estrogen alone or combined HRT.

Endometrium

Unopposed estrogen therapy increases the risk of cancer, which may be reduced by addition of progesterone. Small increase in incidence is seen with those on sequential combined HRT for at least 5 years, whilst those on continuous combined HRT actually show a lower risk of cancer than the population not on any HRT.

Venous Thromboembolism

Evidence suggests a 2–4 fold increase in the risk of VTE in those on systemic HRT. Changes in coagulation pathway, secondary to increase in procoagulant factors are thought to be responsible for this finding. Other nonhormonal factors such as age, BMI, family history of thrombosis, immobility, surgery, and hospitalization further increase the risk. In the presence of strong family history, thrombophilia screening may be offered prior to the initiation of HRT. Transdermal estrogens may be a good alternative in such group of patients at higher risk. Thromboprophylaxis may be considered in those patients at high risk who are already on HRT.

Hormone Replacement Therapy Overview: 2012 Cochrane Collaboration Systemic Review

Cochrane collaboration systemic review assessed 23 randomized, double-blind studies involving HRT in about 42,830 women, 70% of which were from WHI and HERS. Majority of focus being on older menopausal women, not surprisingly, review group found an increased risk of CVD, VTE, breast cancer, stroke, gallbladder disease, and dementia in women >65 years of age. This review also concluded that HRT was not indicated for either primary or secondary prevention of both CVD and dementia. Significant reduction in fractures especially after use of 5 years was seen but however, use of HRT for prevention of postmenopausal osteoporosis was recommended in those only with high risk for fragility fractures and in those presenting with vasomotor symptoms or intolerant for other treatment options.

Hormone Replacement Therapy: Dosage, Routes, and Side Effects

In perimenopausal women who are still menstruating or women who have had at least one menses within the last year, estrogens (estradiol or conjugated estrogen) and progesterone (e.g., norethisterone, MPA, dydrogesterone) may be used as sequential combined regimen that has continuous estrogen combined with 12–14 days of progesterone in the latter half of the cycle. Women with established menopause may be offered continuous combined regimens with both estrogen and progesterone (ethinylestradiol 0.02 mg + levonorgestrel 0.10 mg) which would serve the same purpose but without cyclical monthly bleeds. Ultra low dose estradiol/progesterone (0.5 mg estradiol + 2.5 mg dydrogesterone) used in such continuous combined regimes do help in reducing the side effects, yet retaining the efficacy. Further reduction in side effects could also be achieved by using transdermal patches, gels, and subcutaneous implants of estrogen that can bypass first pass metabolism. Intact uterus warrants the need to supplement progesterone to minimize endometrial hyperplasia and carcinoma. Progesterones can be used in oral micronized forms, vaginal pessaries or gel. The levonorgestrel intrauterine system is now licensed for 4 years, which provides minimal systemic progestogenic side effects due to direct release into the endometrium.

Hormone replacement therapy discontinuation is mostly due to progesterone intolerance with fluid retention, androgenic side effects especially with testosterone derivatives like norethisterone, mood swings, and premenstrual syndrome (PMS) like symptoms and break through bleeding. This can be managed by decreasing the dose and duration of progesterone supplementation. However, whilst managing "break through bleed" which is more common with continuous regimens, one can switch over to sequential regimens instead, if it persists for >3–6 months. If bleed becomes erratic or heavy, doubling the progestogenic dose or increasing its use to 21 days (instead of 14) may also be considered. Any irregular bleed beyond 6 months warrants further investigation with ultrasound and/or an endometrial biopsy.

Various preparations that are commercially available in India with examples are mentioned in appendix (Refer to **Appendix 1**).

CONCLUSION

With menopause, women are likely to not only experience multiple symptoms related to their reproductive life but are also at increased risk of both heart disease and osteoporotic fractures. With increasing lifespan, these issues if not addressed in the right time could cripple their long term health and quality of life. Menopause, hence should be used as an opportunity by the healthcare professionals to explore clinical needs of women and address them appropriately.

SUGGESTED READINGS

1. Khadilkar AV, Mandlik RM. Epidemiology and treatment of osteoporosis in women: an Indian perspective. Int J Womens Health. 2015;7:841-50.
2. Meeta, Harinarayan CV, Marwah R, et al. Clinical practice guidelines on postmenopausal osteoporosis: An executive summary and recommendations. J Midlife Health. 2013;4(2): 107-26.
3. Pachman DR, Jones JM, Loprinzi CL. Management of menopause-associated vasomotor symptoms: Current treatment options, challenges and future directions. Int J Womens Health. 2010;2:123-35.
4. Rossouw JE, Prentice RL, Manson JE, et al. Postmenopausal Hormone Therapy and Risk of Cardiovascular Disease by Age and Years Since Menopause. JAMA. 2007;297(13):1465-77.
5. Shanafelt TD, Barton DL, Adjei AA, et al. Pathophysiology and treatment of hot flashes. Mayo Clin Proc. 2002;77(11):1207-18.

Appendix 1

1. Estrogen formulations

Tablets

Estradiol	1 mg (e.g., Evalon, Progynova)	2 mg (e.g., Evalon, Progynova)	
Conjugated estrogen	0.3 mg (e.g., Premarin)	0.625 mg (e.g., Premarin, Conjugase, Espauz)	1.25 mg (e.g., Premarin)

Patch and pessary

Pessary (daily)	Patch (once in 3–4 days)
E2 (vaginal) 2 mg/1 pessary	• Estraderm MX: 0.025 mg/1 patch, 0.1 mg/1 patch, 1.5 mg/1 patch • ETS 1.8 mg/1 patch

Gels and cream (local application)

Creams	Gels
• Evalon vaginal cream 1 mg/1 g (estradiol) • Premarin VG 0.625 mg/1 m (conjugated estrogen)	• E2 Gel (5 G): 35%, Oestrogel: 3mg/5 g • Sandrena: 1 mg/1 g

ESTROGEN RING: Estradiol vaginal ring; 2 mg/1 ring (90 days)

2. Progesterone formulations

Tablets

Micronized progesterone	100 mg (e.g., Microgest, susten)	200 mg (e.g., Microgest, susten)	400 mg (e.g., Microgest, susten)
Norethisterone	5 mg (e.g., Primolut N)		
Dydrogesterone	10 mg (e.g., Duphaston)	100 mg (e.g., Duphaston)	
Medroxyprogesterone acetate	2.5 mg (e.g., Meprate)	5 mg (e.g., Empeea)	10 mg (e.g., Meprate)

19 Precocious Puberty in Females

CHAPTER

Beatrice Anne M, Chitra Selvan

CASE VIGNETTE

A 5-year-old girl was brought by her mother to her primary care physician with concerns of progressive enlargement of the breasts for the last 3 months. There was no increase in height compared to the peers nor any vaginal bleeding/ appearance of pubic or axillary hair. On examination, the child was in Tanner stage 2 of breast development with no pubic/axillary hair. Her height was in the 75th percentile for age. The vaginal mucosa was pink, indicating no signs of estrogenization. On evaluation, her bone age was around 6 years and uterine volume by ultrasonography was 2.5 mL. Her thyroid function tests were normal. The basal luteinizing hormone (LH) was 1.94 IU/L and follicle-stimulating hormone (FSH) was 2.38 IU/L. There were no signs of increased intracranial tension. Her MRI hypothalamo-pituitary region was normal.

DEFINITION

Sexual precocity is the appearance of any sign of secondary sexual maturation before the lower limit of the normal age of onset of puberty (i.e., 9 years for boys, 7 years for white girls, and 6 years for African-American girls). Just how early is too early has been a matter of debate, as the age of onset of puberty has progressively decreased over the years. Hence, a more prudent way to define sexual precocity will be sex hormone production or exposure occurring earlier than the norms for gender and racial or ethnic background.

NORMAL PUBERTY

To understand the pathophysiology of precocious puberty, it is essential to have an understanding of the physiology of normal puberty. The sequence of events in the normal pubertal development in girls is thelarche (development of breast buds) followed by adrenarche (growth of pubic and axillary hair) and menarche. Thelarche is primarily under the control of estrogens secreted by the ovary and adrenarche is governed by the androgens secreted by the adrenal cortex and ovary. Since these two events are controlled by different endocrine organs, discordance can occur and, hence, the breast and pubic hair developmental stages should be graded separately. In this regard, Tanner staging system is the most widely used. Menarche usually occurs during Tanner stage 4 breast development.

The production of kisspeptin by arcuate nucleus and anteroventral periventricular area of the hypothalamus kick-start the cascade of events in normal puberty. Kisspeptin alters the secretion of gonadotropin-releasing hormone (GnRH) from the hypothalamus, the amplitude and frequency of which are low in a prepubertal child. Neurokinin B and dynorphin from the same neurons stimulate and inhibit the release of kisspeptin, respectively and, hence, these kisspeptin, neurokinin, and dynorphin neurons have now been recognized to be central to puberty initiation. In the early stages of puberty, GnRH pulse amplitude increases and pulse frequency increases to every 1–2 hours, primarily at night. These changes then extend into the day as the puberty progresses. In response to these changes in GnRH secretion, LH and FSH production also increase, initially during the night and then during the day in later pubertal stages. This increase in FSH promotes early follicular development in the ovary and in conjunction with LH leads to gradually increasing estradiol secretion. In early puberty, estrogen levels are low with peaks occurring in the morning hours. These levels increase and are maintained throughout the day as puberty progresses.

CAUSES OF PRECOCIOUS PUBERTY

The causes of precocious puberty can be broadly classified as GnRH dependent and GnRH independent. GnRH-dependent precocious puberty, also referred to as central precocious puberty (CPP), occurs due to premature activation of the hypothalamic-pituitary-gonadal axis due to various pathologic processes involving the central nervous system (CNS). Unlike boys with precocious puberty, where there is more likelihood of identifying a pathology, girls with CPP most commonly do not have any identifiable cause. Idiopathic CPP comprises almost 90% of cases in females. In GnRH-independent precocious puberty, production of sex steroids occurs independent of GnRH, e.g., from ovarian cysts or adrenal tumors.

APPROACH TO THE PATIENT WITH PRECOCIOUS PUBERTY

In precocious puberty, be it GnRH dependent or independent, classically along with the presence of secondary sexual characters, there is a spurt in height velocity and advancement in bone age due to the effect of the gonadal steroids on the skeletal system.

When evaluating a child for sexual precocity, it is essential to differentiate between the variations of pubertal development such as premature thelarche and premature pubarche from sexual precocity.

Premature thelarche is defined as unilateral or bilateral breast enlargement without other signs of sexual maturation (e.g., sexual hair, growth of the labia minora, growth of the uterus). The disorder usually is seen by age 2 years in >80% of cases and rarely after age 4 years. Breast enlargement usually regresses after a few months, but may occasionally persist for years or until the onset of normal puberty. In about half of affected girls, the breast development, which is characteristically cyclic, lasts 3–5 years. This is found with age of onset over 2 years. Long-term follow-up has not shown any untoward effects on later health, growth, or fertility. Although only follow-up and reassurance are required in these cases, it has to be kept in mind that thelarche could be the harbinger of further pubertal maturation in a few cases. But, there are no pointers to predict which of these patients will progress to puberty. Hence, there is a need for careful clinical follow-up (**Table 1**).

TABLE 1: Causes of sexual precocity in females.

GnRH-dependent sexual precocity	GnRH-independent sexual precocity
• Idiopathic true precocious puberty	• Ovarian cyst
• *CNS tumors*:	• Estrogen-secreting ovarian or adrenal neoplasm
○ Optic glioma associated with neurofibromatosis type 1	• Peutz–Jeghers syndrome
○ Hypothalamic astrocytoma	• McCune–Albright syndrome
• *Other CNS disorders*:	• Hypothyroidism
○ Developmental abnormalities including hypothalamic hamartoma of the tuber cinereum	• Iatrogenic or exogenous sexual precocity (including inadvertent exposure to estrogens in food, drugs, or cosmetics)
○ Encephalitis	*Variations of pubertal development*:
○ Static encephalopathy	• Premature thelarche
○ Brain abscess	• Premature isolated menarche
○ Sarcoid or tubercular granuloma	• Premature adrenarche
○ Head trauma	
○ Hydrocephalus	
○ Arachnoid cyst	
○ Myelomeningocele	
○ Vascular lesion	
○ Cranial irradiation	
○ True precocious puberty after late treatment of congenital virilizing adrenal hyperplasia or other previous chronic exposure to sex steroids	
○ True precocious puberty due to gain of function mutations:	
– In *KISS1R/GPR54* gene	
– In *KISS1* gene	

(CNS: central nervous system; GnRH: gonadotropin-releasing hormone; GPR54: G protein-coupled receptor 54; *KISS1R*: kisspeptin)

Source: Modified from Grumbach MM. True or central precocious puberty. In: Kreiger DT, Bardin CW (Eds). Current Therapy in Endocrinology and Metabolism, 1985-1986. Toronto, Canada: BC Decker; 1985. pp. 4-8.

Exaggerated thelarche is described as premature thelarche with the added findings of advanced bone age and increased growth rate, which are estrogen effects. Premature adrenarche (i.e., pubarche) is defined as precocious appearance of pubic hair or axillary hair or both. This is usually associated with an apocrine odor, comedones, and acne, without other signs of puberty or virilization. Premature adrenarche is mostly slowly progressive and does not have an untoward effect on either the onset or the normal progression of gonadarche or final adult height. It may be considered to be a normal variation in the differentiation, growth, and function of the zona reticularis of the adrenal cortex, marked biochemically by the precocious increase in the concentration of plasma dehydroepiandrosterone sulfate (DHEAS) to >40 µg/dL and is developmentally regulated. The studies have shown that girls with premature adrenarche are at increased risk of developing functional ovarian hyperandrogenism and polycystic ovary syndrome (PCOS), hyperinsulinism, and dyslipidemia in adolescence and adult life, especially if fetal growth was reduced and the birth weight was low. The differential diagnosis includes nonclassic 21-hydroxylase and 11β-hydroxylase deficiencies.

Once sexual precocity has been established, the next step is to distinguish between GnRH-dependent and GnRH-independent causes. A detailed history and a targeted clinical examination are of utmost importance in this scenario. History should be taken from a reliable source (preferably the mother) and should cover the following points:

- Onset and progression of symptoms to assess the tempo of events
- Perinatal events
- Previous infections
- Adventitious ingestion or exposure to gonadal steroids (foods/drugs/cosmetics)
- Gelastic seizures (hypothalamic hamartoma)
- Head trauma
- Cranial irradiation
- Vomiting and seizures (increased intracranial tension due to CNS tumors)

The physical examination should be done in the presence of an unrelated chaperone and should include the following:

- Anthropometry to determine height percentiles and if previous measurements are available, the height velocity to be documented
- Description of the secondary sexual development according to Tanner stages and measurement of the breast tissue in girls (areolar and glandular diameters)
- Examination for comedones and acne, oily skin, facial and body hair, pubic and axillary hair development, axillary apocrine gland odor, and galactorrhea
- Examination of the external genitalia to look for dulling and thickening of the vaginal mucosa and enlargement of the labia minora

- Goiter and signs of hypothyroidism
- Neurologic examination with emphasis on assessment of the visual fields and optic disks in search for signs of increased intracranial pressure
- Evaluation for skin lesions associated with the McCune–Albright syndrome or neurofibromatosis (café au lait spots, neurofibromas, Lisch nodules in iris, and axillary freckling)
- Examination for abdominal and adnexal masses

Investigations should include the following:
- Thyroid function tests
- X-rays for determining bone age
- Ultrasonography of the uterus and ovaries
- This step helps to ascertain objectively the effect of estrogen alone, but will not differentiate between GnRH-dependent and -independent causes
  - The upper limit of uterine length in the prepubertal state is 3.5 cm. A uterine volume of >1.8 mL is specific for the onset of puberty, but increased ovarian volume is less specific. The ellipsoid volume of the uterus is calculated by V = longitudinal diameter × anteroposterior diameter × transverse diameter × 0.523. The presence of an endometrial stripe is indicative of precocious puberty. Cysts may be found in the ovaries in patients with CPP or GnRH-independent isosexual precocity; they usually are smaller than 9 mm in the former and larger than 9 mm in the latter.
- LH, FSH, estradiol, and LH response to GnRH agonist
- The principle behind this test is that in GnRH-dependent causes of precocious puberty, when GnRH is injected, there is an exaggerated rise in LH
  - A recent study stated that patients with a basal LH level of 0.3 IU/L or higher had subsequent pubertal progression, whereas 39 of 41 patients with a basal LH level of 0.2 IU/L or lower did not progress. Triptorelin (100 μg) and leuprolide (20 μg/m²) are the most commonly available GnRH agonist for GnRH agonist stimulation test in India. These preparations are usually administered subcutaneous or intramuscular (IM). The prepubertal upper limit of normal for basal LH, determined by the 95th percentile of the prepubertal population, was 0.2 IU/L [immunochemiluminometric assay (ICMA)] and 0.6 IU/L [immunofluorometric assay (IFMA)]. The LH peak after GnRH stimulation that defined puberty was 3.3 IU/L (ICMA) and 4.2 IU/L (IFMA) in girls. The interpretation of these tests in the various clinical settings is elaborated in **Table 2**.

Other relevant investigations will include:
- *MRI of the hypothalamic-pituitary region*: The primary goal is rule out the presence of any CNS tumors/mass that could have caused the CPP. The height of the pituitary gland on MRI correlates with advancing age

TABLE 2: Differential diagnosis of sexual precocity.

Disorders	Plasma gonadotropins	LH response to GnRH	Serum sex steroid concentration
True precocious puberty	Prominent LH pulses (premature reactivation of GnRH pulse generator)	Pubertal LH response initially during sleep	Pubertal values of estradiol
Granulosa cell tumor (follicular cysts may present similarly)	Suppressed	Prepubertal LH response	Very high estradiol
Follicular cyst	Suppressed	Prepubertal LH response	Prepubertal to very high estradiol
Feminizing adrenal tumor	Suppressed	Prepubertal LH response	High estradiol and DHEAS values
Premature thelarche	Prepubertal	Prepubertal and pubertal LH response	Prepubertal or early estradiol response
Premature adrenarche	Prepubertal	Prepubertal LH response	Prepubertal estradiol; DHEAS or urinary 17-ketosteroid values appropriate for pubic hair stage 2
Late-onset virilizing congenital adrenal hyperplasia	Prepubertal	Prepubertal LH response	Elevated 17-OHP in basal or corticotropin-stimulated state
McCune–Albright syndrome	Suppressed	Suppressed	Sex steroid pubertal or higher
Primary hypothyroidism	LH prepubertal; FSH may be slightly elevated	Prepubertal FSH may be increased	Estradiol may be pubertal

(DHEAS: dehydroepiandrosterone sulfate; FSH: follicle-stimulating hormone; GnRH: gonadotropin-releasing hormone; LH: luteinizing hormone; 17-OHP: 17-hydroxyprogesterone)

and with pubertal development. Those patients with CPP had pituitary heights exceeding 6 mm on average, whereas those with precocious thelarche had lower heights. The shape of the pituitary gland is also of importance: A convex appearance rather than a flat top is associated with CPP of any cause. But, neither the size nor the shape of the pituitary gland decreases with successful GnRH therapy

- Skeletal survey (McCune–Albright syndrome)
- Imaging of abdomen (if adrenal tumor suspected)
- 17-hydroxyprogesterone [if late-onset congenital adrenal hyperplasia (CAH) suspected]
- Anti-Müllerian hormone (AMH) and inhibin (in case of granulosa cell tumors causing sexual precocity)

TREATMENT

The drugs used in the management of true precocious puberty are:
- Medroxyprogesterone acetate (MPA)
- Cyproterone acetate (CPA)
- GnRH agonists

Medroxyprogesterone Acetate

Medroxyprogesterone acetate inhibits gonadotropin secretion by its action on the hypothalamic GnRH pulse generator/pituitary gonadotropin unit and exerts a direct suppressive effect on gonadal steroidogenesis through 3β-hydroxysteroid dehydrogenase 2 (3β-HSD2). The adverse effects of MPA occur due to its glucocorticoid action, which can suppress adreno-corticotropic hormone (ACTH) and cortisol secretion, increase appetite and lead to excessive weight gain, and can induce hypertension and a cushingoid appearance.

Dosing

10 mg once a day orally/MPA depot deep IM injections, at a low dose of 50 mg per month, which can be increased up to 400 mg per month or the dosing frequency can be reduced to fortnightly.

Cyproterone Acetate

Cyproterone acetate has antiandrogenic, antigonadotropic, and progesta-tional properties. It suppresses the secretion of ACTH and the plasma concentration of cortisol. Secondary adrenal insufficiency can cause fatigue and weakness. In contrast to MPA, this agent lacks gluconeogenic activity and does not appear to produce cushingoid features. The use of both these drugs has been replaced by the more efficacious GnRH agonists, but they can be used as second-line drugs for the occasional patient who cannot tolerate GnRH agonists due to untoward effects.

Gonadotropin-releasing Hormone Agonists

The treatment of choice for CPP is the GnRH agonists, synthetic analogs of the amino acid sequence of the natural GnRH decapeptide. The agonist binds to the GnRH receptor on gonadotrophs, which leads to desensitization of the gonadotroph to GnRH and downregulation and loss of receptors. Desensitization persists after receptor levels return to normal as a result of uncoupling of the receptors from the intracellular signaling effector pathway. This mechanism of action produces a form of reversible medical gonadectomy. Every 4-week and every 12-week formulations of leuprorelin (leuprolide acetate) have been Food and Drug Administration (FDA) approved for the treatment of CPP. Depot leuprolide acetate, GnRH analog, consists of leuprolide enclosed in microspheres of a glycolic and lactic acid copolymer, which causes its slow release. The free leuprolide is also present in the preparation and is absorbed into the circulation within minutes following injection. A subcutaneous implant of histrelin was approved for 12-month treatment of CPP and recent studies show efficacy for 2 years before removal is necessary. Treatment of CPP with a potent GnRH agonist results in a transient increased FSH and LH release for 1–3 days and a rise in circulating gonadal steroid levels, followed after 7–14 days of treatment by suppression of pulsatile secretion of LH and FSH and of the pubertal LH response to the administration of native GnRH. A plasma estradiol concentration of <18 pmol/L (5 pg/mL) in girls indicates adequate gonadal suppression and this takes about 2–4 weeks in girls. GnRH agonist therapy does not affect the secretion of adrenal androgens. The major conclusions of the International Consensus Conference convened by the Lawson Wilkins Pediatric Endocrine Society and the European Society for Pediatric Endocrinology to review the use of GnRH were as follows:

- GnRH analogs exert benefit in increasing adult height in children with early-onset CPP (<6 years in girls) and are not routinely recommended after that age
- The alteration of psychosocial effects of CPP by GnRH analogs requires additional study
- The use of GnRH analogs does not lead to weight gain or long-term diminution of bone mineral density (BMD)
- The use of GnRH analogs for conditions other than CPP, such as to increase adult height in children with idiopathic short stature or small for gestational age (SGA) or with growth hormone (GH) treatment in children, is not recommended

Dosing

Gonadotropin-releasing hormone agonist injections can be given monthly or once in 3 months.

With the 1-month depot, it has been shown that 3.75 mg injections (roughly 120 µg/kg) are efficient in almost all children with CPP. The commonly recommended dose for the 1-month depot contrasts between the European Union (3.75 mg or 120 µg/kg) and the United States (300 µg/kg). The minimum effective dose in children has been shown to be 30 µg/kg. Several randomized studies have shown an equivalence between the 1-month and 3-month preparations at the respective doses of 3.75 and 11.25 mg (**Table 3**). Leuprorelin 3-month depot has been shown to efficiently inhibit the pituitary-gonadal axis in 95% of children studied with CPP during a 6-month trial. In girls, estradiol levels were more rapidly and uniformly suppressed with the 3-month depot than with the 1-month depot. Long-term studies are required to assess the efficacy of the 3-month depot preparation. The first injection of GnRH agonist is associated with a transient surge in LH and FSH resulting in a transient increase in estradiol levels, which then rapidly reduces following downregulation of GnRH receptor, usually within

TABLE 3: GnRH agonists preparations available in India.

Agents	Preparations available
Leuprolide	• 3.75 mg monthly IM • 11.25 mg 3 monthly IM
Triptorelin	• 3.75 mg monthly IM • 11.25 mg 3 monthly IM
Goserelin	10.8 mg 3 monthly (available as subcutaneous implant)

(GnRH: gonadotropin-releasing hormone; IM: intramuscular)

a fortnight. The transient surge in estradiol may result in vaginal spotting/bleeding in a small fraction of female patients following the first injection. Hence, it may be important to counsel the parents about this possibility to allay any undue anxiety. Depot MPA can be coinjected only with the first dose of GnRH agonist that may be a reasonable option to prevent this estradiol surge and the associated vaginal bleed.

The adverse reactions seen with GnRH agonist therapy are:
- Local and systemic allergic reactions
- Sterile abscess in the injection site
- Slipped capital epiphyses occur mostly during the earliest phase of puberty, when growth is beginning to increase, and not after fusion of the triradiate cartilage, so the few cases reported after GnRH agonist treatment may have a different etiologic course than that found in average pubertal children.

Autonomously functioning ovarian follicular cysts, presenting as precocious puberty, can be treated with oral MPA, which seems to prevent recurrence, to accelerate involution of the follicular cysts, and to reduce the risk of torsion. Another potential approach is the use of a potent aromatase inhibitor such as letrozole to reduce estradiol secretion. This approach has proved successful in McCune–Albright syndrome, which may present solely with autonomous ovarian cysts with no other stigmata. A recently published clinical trial of fulvestrant, a pure estrogen receptor blocker, has shown promising results. Surgical intervention is rarely indicated; a large or persistent cyst can be reduced by puncture at laparoscopy and the size of the cyst can be monitored readily by pelvic sonography. MPA has been associated with regression of the cysts in estradiol-secreting ovarian cysts occurring in preterm infants born before 30 weeks of gestation, even though the LH and FSH response to GnRH in these patients suggests GnRH dependence.

Another important aspect of management of precocious puberty is the psychosocial issues related to the early onset of puberty in the affected girls as well as the parents. The affected child might become a subject of peer ridicule due to the advanced physical development and the child may seek friends closer to her size and physical development. Sex education of the child and the family is essential and must be given in a skillful, sensitive, and explicit manner; the risks of sexual abuse and of pregnancy need to be discussed. The parents as well as the child need to be educated about the management of menses. There might be discrepancies between the child's mental, physical, and psychosexual development and the unrealistic expectations and demands from the society may add onto these problems. These have to be dealt in a very sensitive manner.

MONITORING AND FOLLOW-UP

Changes in secondary sexual characteristics seen within the first 6 months of therapy include reduction in breast size and decrease in pubic hair, cessation of menses, if present before treatment, and decreased size of the uterus and ovaries as assessed by pelvic sonography in girls. Some girls may experience recurrent episodes of hot flushes and moodiness. Height velocity has been shown to decrease by about 60% during the first year of therapy, with greater decrease found in those with the most advanced bone age and taller relative height at the start of treatment. The lowest growth velocities are seen in longer duration of puberty before treatment, the most advanced physical findings, and the most rapid bone age advancement before therapy. The best height advantage can be obtained when treatment is begun soon after the onset of precocity and when the bone age is advanced by only a few years.

Follow-up visits should be done at more frequent intervals of 1–3 months at the start of therapy and the following parameters should be monitored:
• Height velocity
• Regression of secondary sexual characters
• Serial evaluation of ovarian morphologic appearance and uterine size by pelvic ultrasonography
• LH response to exogenous GnRH agonists
• Bone age by appropriate X-rays
   The advantage of hormonal evaluation over clinical parameters during therapy with GnRH analog is a timely correction of the depot leuprolide dose can be done, avoiding pubertal advancement and finally shorter height.
   The LH response to a GnRH test is the most convincing way to determine sufficient hypothalamic-pituitary-gonadal axis suppression. A complete standard test may not always be necessary. Several studies have sought alternative means of evaluating LH suppression in children receiving GnRH analog therapy. A single LH sample 40 minutes after subcutaneous GnRH, overnight LH values, 24-hour urinary gonadotropin excretion, and a single plasma estradiol measurement 12 hours after an IM injection of a GnRH agonist have been studied as simpler parameters for monitoring. A peak LH cutoff value of <3.3 IU/L, 3 hours after depot leuprolide injection, may be used as an indicator of adequate LH suppression.

RESUMPTION OF NORMAL PUBERTY AND LONG-TERM OUTCOMES

The reversal of gonadal suppression happens within a few weeks to months, as manifested by a rise in the concentration of plasma gonadal steroids, progression of sexual maturation, and return of menses. Treatment is to be continued till 10 years of age in girls and a history of peers' pubertal status and achievement of menarche should be noted, so that the treatment can be stopped accordingly. Menarche occurs at an average of 1.2–1.5 years after discontinuation of therapy (range: 0–60 months). Ovulation happens in 50% of girls by 1 year after menarche and in 90% of those studied 2 or more years after menarche and pregnancies have been reported in GnRH agonist-treated girls. In a follow-up study of 47 patients treated for precocious puberty, there was no difference in the incidence of menstrual irregularity, significant dysmenorrhea, number of pregnancies, or pregnancy outcome.

Adult height in children treated with GnRH agonists is improved, especially when therapy starts before 6 years of age rather than after 8 years of age. In a study of 87 girls with idiopathic gonadotropin-dependent precocious puberty, GnRH analog treatment for 3–8 years was associated with adult height being 9.5 ± 4.6 cm higher than the predicted adult height at the onset of treatment. Similar findings were observed in an Indian study of 30 girls with gonadotropin-dependent precocious puberty treated with GnRH analog, triptorelin was given for a mean period of 3.7 years where a height gain of 6.4 cm compared to pretreatment predicted adult height was seen. The predictors of good height outcomes include younger chronological age, younger bone age, greater height standard deviation score for chronological age at initiation of therapy, and a higher predicted adult height using Bayley–Pinneau tables. The addition of human GH treatment to the GnRH regimen can be considered when growth velocity is reduced sufficiently over a 6-month period to compromise predicted final height, but must be considered experimental. Peak bone mass or body composition will not be impaired in patients with precocious puberty after GnRH agonist therapy. Calcium and vitamin D intake must be ensured during treatment to achieve optimal skeletal health. MPA/CPA is useful in halting puberty progression, but has no beneficial impact on final height outcomes.

Girls with CPP have a tendency toward obesity that is unrelated to treatment with GnRH agonist. An increased prevalence of PCOS has been noted in young women (mean age: 18.1 years) with a history of CPP, with onset at a mean age of 7.65 years. However, this finding is controversial as different criteria have been used in various studies with lack of adequate controls. CPP in females does not lead to premature menopause. However, there is increased risk in girls for the development of carcinoma of the breast in adulthood.

CONCLUSION

Coming back to the clinical problem, the abovementioned patient had presented with sexual precocity at the age of 5 years. The physician made a diagnosis of idiopathic GnRH-dependent precocious puberty. In this case, thelarche was the presenting feature of the complete isosexual precocious puberty. She was started on GnRH agonist (injection leuprolide 3.75 mg) monthly injections. After 3 months, after the start of treatment, her basal LH level came down to 0.1 IU/L, 3 hours post-GnRH injection LH was 1.2 IU/L, and the uterine volume was 1.4 mL. The patient should be under regular follow-up and the treatment should be withdrawn at 10 or 11 years, at an age commiserate with the onset of menarche in her peers.

SUGGESTED READINGS

1. Aguirre RS, Eugster EA. Central precocious puberty: From genetics to treatment. Best Pract Res Clin Endocrinol Metab. 2018;32(4):343-54.
2. Bridges NA, Cooke A, Healy MJ, Hindmarsh PC, Brook CG. Ovaries in sexual precocity. Clin Endocrinol (Oxf). 1995;42:135-40.
3. Carel JC, Léger J. Clinical practice. Precocious puberty. N Engl J Med. 2008;358(22):2366-77
4. de Vries L, Guz-Mark A, Lazar L, Reches A, Phillip M. Premature thelarche: age at presentation affects clinical course but not clinical characteristics or risk to progress to precocious puberty. J Pediatr. 2010;156:466-71.
5. de Vries L, Horev G, Schwartz M, Phillip M. Ultrasonographic and clinical parameters for early differentiation between precocious puberty and premature thelarche. Eur J Endocrinol. 2006;154:891-8.
6. Grumbach MM, Richards GE, Conte FA, Kaplan SL. Clinical disorders of adrenal function and puberty: an assessment of the role of the adrenal cortex in normal and abnormal puberty in man and evidence for an ACTH-like pituitary adrenal androgen-stimulating hormone. In: James VHT, Serio M, Giusti G, Martini L (Eds). The Endocrine Function of the Human Adrenal Cortex. New York: Academic Press; 1978. pp. 583-612.
7. Harrington J, Palmert MR, Hamilton J. Use of local data to enhance uptake of published recommendations: an example from the diagnostic evaluation of precocious puberty. Arch Dis Child. 2014;99:15-20
8. Latronico AC, Brito VN, Carel JC. Causes, diagnosis, and treatment of central precocious puberty. Lancet Diabetes Endocrinol. 2016;4(3):265-74.
9. Melmed S, Polonsky K, Larsen PR, Kronenberg H. William's Textbook of Endocrinology, 13th edition. New York: Elsevier; 2015.
10. Soriano-Guillén L, Argente J. Central precocious puberty, functional and tumor-related. Best Pract Res Clin Endocrinol Metab. 2019;33(3):101262.
11. Van Winter JT, Noller KL, Zimmerman D, Melton LJ. Natural history of premature thelarche in Olmsted County, Minnesota, 1940 to 1984. J Pediatr. 1990;116:278-80.
12. Volta C, Bernasconi S, Cisternino M, Buzi F, Ferzetti A, Street ME, et al. Isolated premature thelarche and thelarche variant: clinical and auxological follow-up of 119 girls. J Endocrinol Invest. 1998;21:180-3.

20

CHAPTER

Primary Ovarian Insufficiency

PG Sundararaman, Chandar Mohan Batra

INTRODUCTION

Primary ovarian insufficiency (POI) is defined as the loss of ovarian function before 40 years of age, characterized by amenorrhea (primary or secondary) (>4 months) with raised gonadotropins in the postmenopausal range [follicle-stimulating hormone (FSH)] >30–40 mIU/mL], and low estradiol. There should be two serum FSH levels obtained at least 1 month apart in the menopausal range. Previously, this condition was also called premature menopause, premature ovarian failure (POF), primary ovarian failure, hypergonadotropic hypogonadism, and gonadal dysgenesis till an American consensus meeting in 2009 named the condition as POI. The prevalence is 1 in 10,000 women by the age of 20 years, 1 in 1,000 women by the age of 30 years, and 1 in 100 women by the age of 40 years. The familial form of POF is rare, representing 4–31% of all cases of POF.

Primary ovarian insufficiency occurs through two major mechanisms: Follicle dysfunction and follicle depletion. There is either an inadequate initial pool of follicles or an acceleration of destruction of follicles by an autoimmune or toxic mechanism. Follicles may be present in the ovary but may not be able to function due to some mechanism, probably genetic.

The causes of POI are genetic, autoimmune, ovarian surgery, cytotoxic cancer therapy, metabolic and storage disorders, and infections.

The clinical picture is subtle, with reduced energy, primary or secondary amenorrhea, decreased sex drive, psychological insults, and hot flushes. This disease is associated with infertility and an increased risk of osteoporosis, cardiovascular diseases, and early mortality. POI is variable in its clinical presentation. Amenorrhea is secondary in 84% cases and primary in 16% cases. Age of onset varies from puberty to 40 years. Women with primary amenorrhea have an earlier age of onset of symptoms and breast and pubertal development is incomplete in 70% cases whereas, those with secondary amenorrhea have a later age of onset and pubertal development is complete. POI can be permanent or transient. Spontaneous subsequent ovulation cycles can occur in 25% and some (4.4%) may even conceive.

POI may also be associated with other autoimmune disorders, the dry eye syndrome (Sjögren's disease), myasthenia gravis, rheumatoid arthritis, systemic lupus erythematosus (SLE) and Hashimoto thyroiditis, so hyperpigmentation, vitiligo, puffy face, dry skin, goiter, exophthalmos, and rash have to be looked for.

A family history of the fragile X syndrome, intellectual disability, dementia, tremor or ataxia, or symptoms similar to those associated with Parkinson's disease might point to a premutation in the fragile X mental retardation 1 (*FMR1*) gene, as a cause of POI.

Primary ovarian insufficiency may be syndromic with other features such as impaired hearing in Perrault syndrome, eyelid abnormalities in blepharophimosis/ptosis/epicanthus inversus syndrome (BPES), cerebellar dysfunction in ataxia telangiectasia, or short stature in Turner syndrome.

The cause remains unknown in 65% of the patients despite extensive investigation, which is labeled as idiopathic.

CASE HISTORY

Ms SN, a 28-year-old unmarried woman, presented with a 13 months' amenorrhea. She attained her menarche at the age of 13 years. Amenorrhea was preceded by oligomenorrhea followed by irregular menses, which responded to progesterone withdrawal bleed initially. She also complained of hot flashes, night sweats, and decreased libido. There was no family history of irregular menses. Patient did not have history of diabetes mellitus, hypothyroidism, rheumatoid arthritis, kidney disease, ataxia, tremors, or excessive exercise. There was no history of intake of drugs for any other disease, oral contraceptive use, or anticancer drugs. There was no history of excessive weight gain, striae, hirsutism, dark patches in axilla, neck, or groin. There was no family history of infertility, irregular menses or premature amenorrhea, malignancy or congenital disorders. She was the product of a nonconsanguineous marriage. She did not smoke or drink alcohol. There was no history of exposure to radiation. Medroxyprogesterone acetate 10 mg daily for 10 days was given after ruling out pregnancy. She had no withdrawal bleed.

She was 165 cm tall and weighed 66 kg; body mass index (BMI) was 23.2 kg/m^2 without any obvious skeletal defects. Thyroid was just palpable. There was no vitiligo, hirsutism, hyperpigmentation, or dry skin. Axillary hair were normal, breasts were Tanner stage 5 without galactorrhea, and clitoromegaly was not present. Routine clinical evaluation including anthropometric measurement and system examination was normal. There was no webbing of neck, short stature or stigmata indicative of Turner syndrome. Her hearing was normal; no cerebellar signs or eyelid abnormalities were present. No other congenital malformations were detected and the systemic examination was within normal limits. Her IQ was normal and there was no focal neurological deficit.

Investigations

Her routine hematological and biochemical tests were normal. Her hormonal tests were as follows:

- Serum calcium: 8.8 mg/dL
- Phosphorous: 4.6 mg/dL
- Alkaline phosphatase: 20 units/L
- 25-hydroxy vitamin D: 20 ng/mL (>30)
- Parathyroid hormone (PTH): 80 pg/mL
- TSH: 3.12 µ/mL (0.4–4.2)
- Anti-thyroid peroxidase (Anti-TPO) antibodies: Negative
- Prolactin (PRL): 12.4 ng/mL (2–29)
- FSH: 48 mIU/mL (3–20)
- Luteinizing hormone (LH): 37 mIU/mL (5–25)
- Estradiol 12 pg/mL (25–75)
- Serum cortisol: 20 µg/dL (8 AM), 8 µg/dL (4 PM)
- Ultrasound pelvis: Normal-sized uterus, right ovary volume 2 cc, left ovary volume 4 cc, normal stroma, endometrial thickness measuring 0.8 mm, and no follicles seen
- Karyotype: 46,XX
- Ovarian biopsy was not done
- Dual energy X-ray absorptiometry) scan: T Score—1.0 spine
- T score—0.8 hip
- Anti-Müllerian hormone (AMH) was nondetectable

Diagnosis

- Premature ovarian insufficiency; cause—idiopathic
- Vitamin D deficiency
- Mild osteopenia

Management

In addition to hormone replacement, she was started on calcium and vitamin D supplements. Psychological counseling was given. She is having periodic monitoring of health status. She was counseled that she still had 5–10% chances of having spontaneous menstrual periods and pregnancy. If she wanted pregnancy, the options available to her were adoption, in vitro fertilization (IVF) with donated oocyte or embryo.

Pharmacological Treatment

Estradiol transdermal 100 µg daily from 1st to 21st of every month till the age of 50 years.

Tablet medroxyprogesterone acetate 10 mg from 11th to 21st every month till the age of 50 years.

Tablet calcium carbonate 500 mg twice daily.

Calcirol (vitamin D3) 60,000 units weekly for 8 weeks followed by 60,000 units monthly.

Discussion

This 28-year-old unmarried female presented with secondary amenorrhea following 1 year of irregular periods and typical symptoms of estrogen deficiency.

The most common cause is pregnancy and this should always be excluded even if the patient denies any history of sexual activity. In our case, the ultrasound pelvis was negative for pregnancy. Her ultrasound was negative for polycystic ovarian disease and there was no feature of hyperandrogenism such as hirsutism, acanthosis nigricans or clitomegaly or striae ruling out polycystic ovarian disease, adrenal or ovarian tumor or disorders of sexual differentiation (DSD) as a cause of amenorrhea. The patient's thyroid profile was normal and the patients hematological, biochemical, and radiological profile ruled out any other systemic disorders which can cause amenorrhea. The LH and FSH are high with low estradiol and a normal prolactin which tells us that she had hypergonadotropic hypogonadism due to primary ovarian defect and rules out pituitary and hypothalamic defects.

The karyotype was 46,XX was normal and we did not screen for the *FMR1* gene as we did not have the facilities for this test. The most common genetic abnormalities in this disease are abnormalities in X chromosome that can be a classical Turner 45/XO or a Turner mosaic or permutation of *FMR1* gene. Heredity does play a role although the exact nature of involvement is not yet absolutely clear. Certain genes which run in a woman's family may predispose her to premature menopause. The most common genetic contributor to POI is permutation of *FMR1* gene. This explains 13% of familial cases and 3% of sporadic cases of POI. About 20% of women who carry this permutation of this gene have POI compared to 1% of the general population. *FMR1* gene (Xq27.3) mutations or premutations are typically associated with secondary amenorrhea in female relatives of male patients with mental retardation. Fragile X syndrome is due to CGG expansion (>55 repeats) at the 5'UTR of *FMR1* gene (Xq27.3). The expansion of CGG repeats is associated with gene silencing resulting in male mental retardation and in POI with secondary amenorrhea in female carriers.

Our patient did not have a positive family history of amenorrhea. A positive family history can be a clue to the possibility of *FMR1* premutation or a polyglandular autoimmune syndrome due to a mutation in the *AIRE* gene. It is interesting to note that a positive family history also points to the higher possibility of remission of ovarian insufficiency with ovulation and even pregnancy as compared to those without any positive family history.

Autoimmune oophoritis is responsible for 30% of POI. Other autoimmune disorders such as SLE and Hashimoto's thyroiditis are often found in patients of POI.

Autoimmune adrenalitis can occur with POI and adrenal antibodies against 21OH and 17OH enzymes are positive in many. Our patient did not have any clinical feature of an autoimmune disease and anti-TPO antibodies were negative. Anti-ovarian antibodies are present in some patients of POI but so far they have not been found to be specific and so are not used as a diagnostic or prognostic marker. POI may be part of the autoimmune polyglandular syndromes (APS) when accompanied by other autoimmune endocrinopathies. POI is more common with APS types I and III than with APS type II.

Ovarian biopsy was not done in our patient. It has been noted that ovarian biopsy does not give any conclusive information regarding the etiology of POI or contribute to the management of POI.

Ultrasonography can show two different patterns. Most common is small ovaries with absent follicles and less frequently ovaries of normal surface area with the presence of follicles. The second pattern is associated with higher estradiol and inhibin B pattern. In our patient, the ovaries were small with absent follicles.

Anti-Müllerian hormone is the most reliable tool for diagnosis of POI. It is valuable in assessing ovarian reserve before and after chemotherapy for young women with cancer, before and after ovarian surgery, and for females at high risk of POI. It is accurate and testing can be done in any phase of the menstrual cycle. In our case, it was undetectable.

Inhibin B is another useful marker but it has to be done in the follicular phase of the cycle and has proved to be less reliable than AMH.

We made a diagnosis of POI, cause—idiopathic with vitamin D deficiency and secondary hyperparathyroidism and started the treatment accordingly.

All patients with POI are estrogen deficient. Estrogen has to be replaced from 12 years of age to induce puberty, development of secondary sexual characteristics, preservation of bone health and cardiovascular health, libido, and sexual activity. At the age of 12 years, estrogen supplementation is started at a very small dose of 0.3 mg conjugated estrogen for 6 months and then increased to 0.625 mg of conjugated estrogen for 6 months. Thereafter, conjugated estrogen 0.625 mg daily is given for 21 days every month and medroxyprogesterone acetate is added in a dose of 10 mg daily from 11th to 21st day. This induces cyclical monthly menstrual bleeding.

As a long-term therapy, transdermal estradiol has been found to be equivalent in efficacy and the side effects of oral estrogens such as thrombo-embolism, breast cancer, and endometrial hyperplasia are much less in transdermal estrogens. Our patient was a 28-year-old girl with fully developed secondary sexual characteristics. She was started on transdermal estradiol 100 µg daily for 21 days every month and 10 mg medroxyprogesterone acetate from day 11 to 21.

Bone health of these patients should always be assessed as it is effected by long-term estrogen deficiency. In our patient the calcium, phosphorous, alkaline phosphatase, 25-hydroxy vitamin D, PTH, and a DEXA scan of hips and spine were done. The tests showed vitamin D deficiency, mild osteopenia, and secondary hyperparathyroidism. She was managed with vitamin D and calcium supplementation.

The patient and her parents were educated about POI. They were told about the 10% chance of remission of disease, the use of contraception if sexually active and continuous use of estrogen/progesterone therapy till 50 years of age.

They were told that the patient could get married, have a normal sexual life but would not be able to have children without IVF with donor oocyte or embryo. She was also sent to a psychologist for counseling.

NEW DEVELOPMENTS IN TREATMENT OF PRIMARY OVARIAN INSUFFICIENCY

Techniques of IVF with donor oocyte or embryo have been refined and are highly successful. Stem cell therapy has been tried and one successful pregnancy has been reported. Ovarian transplantation has been found to be successful and implantation of cryopreserved ovarian tissue has been found to be successful.

The most successful infertility treatment has been assisted conception with donated oocytes. Embryo cryopreservation, ovarian tissue or oocyte cryopreservation, and in vitro maturation of oocytes hold promise in cases where ovarian failure is foreseeable as in women undergoing cancer treatments. Thus, the main obstacle in the treatment of POI which was the inability to have children has been overcome.

CONCLUSION

Premature ovarian insufficiency is a fascinating disease. Recent developments have clarified the etiology, diagnosis, treatment, and management of this disease have made it much easier and satisfying to treat. Our ability to give these women children now is an encouraging development in the management of this disease.

SUGGESTED READINGS

1. Beck-Peccoz P, Persani L. Premature ovarian failure. Orphanet J Rare Dis. 2006;1:9.
2. Bidet M, Bachelot A, Bissauge E, Golmard JL, Gricourt S, Dulon J, et al. Resumption of ovarian function and pregnancies in 358 patients with premature ovarian failure. J Clin Endocrinol Metab. 2011;96(12):3864-72.
3. Callejo J, Salvador C, Miralles A, Vilaseca S, Lailla J M, Balasch J. Long-term ovarian function evaluation after autografting by implantation with fresh and frozen thawed human ovarian tissue. Clin Endocrinol Metab. 2001;86(9):4489-94.
4. Chen L, Guo S, Wei C, Li H, Wang H, Xu Y. Effect of stem cell transplantation of premature ovarian failure in animal models and patients: A meta-analysis and case report. Exp Ther Med. 2018;15(5):4105-18.
5. Goswami D, Conway GS. Premature Ovarian Failure. Horm Res. 2007;68:196-202.

6. Hernández-Angeles C, Castelo-Branco C. Early menopause: A hazard to a woman's health. Indian J Med Res. 2016;143(4):420-7.
7. Hormone replacement therapy in young women with primary ovarian insufficiency and early menopause Shannon D. Sullivan; Fertil Steril. 2016;106(7): 1588-99.
8. Jankowska K. Premature ovarian failure. Menopause Rev. 2017;16(2):51-6.
9. Jiao X, Zhang H, Ke H, Zhang J, Cheng L, Liu Y, et al. Premature ovarian insufficiency: Phenotypic characterization within different etiologies. J Clin Endocrinol Metab. 2017;102(7):2281-90.
10. Knauff EAH, Eijkemans MAJ, Lambalk CB, Kate-Booij MJ, Hoek A, Beerendonk CCM. Anti-Mullerian Hormone, Inhibin B, and Antral Follicle Count in Young Women with Ovarian Failure. J Clin Endocrinol Metab. 2009;94(3):786-92.
11. Lunding SA, Aksglaede L, Anderson RA, Main KM, Juul A, Hagen CP, et al. AMH as a predictor of premature ovarian insufficiency: A longitudinal study of 120 Turner syndrome patients. J Clin Endocrinol Metab. 2015;100(7):E1030-8.
12. Ovarian function and reproductive outcome after ovarian tissue transplantation: a systematic review. J Transl Med. 2019;17(1):396.
13. Webber L, Anderson RA, Davies M, Janse F, Vermeulen N. HRT for women with premature ovarian insufficiency: a comprehensive review. Hum Reprod Open. 2017;2017(2):hox007.

21
CHAPTER

Approach to a Patient with Polycystic Ovary Syndrome

Uttio Gupta, Semanti Chakarborty, Shahid Khan,
Mohd Ashraf Ganie, PG Sundararaman

INTRODUCTION

Polycystic ovary syndrome (PCOS) is a widespread and prevalent disorder in women in their reproductive age group and affects 5–10% of that population. The disorder clinically presents as obesity, hirsutism, menstrual disturbances, acne, male pattern baldness, recurrent abortions, infertility, anovulation, and psychological and psychosexual disturbances. In India, prevalence of PCOS ranges between 2.2 and 26% and most of them are overweight or obese.

Three groups have offered diagnostic criteria for PCOS: (1) The National Institutes of Health/National Institute of Child Health and Human Development (NIH/NICHD), (2) The European Society of Human Reproduction and Embryology/American Society for Reproductive Medicine (ESHRE/ASRM), and (3) The Androgen Excess Society (AES).

The AES met in 2006 and debated the merits and demerits of the NIH and the Rotterdam criteria and came up with a practical definition that combines both the PCOS diagnosis criteria. The criteria include all the following: (1) Hyperandrogenism: Hirsutism and/or hyperandrogenemia, (2) Ovarian dysfunction: Oligoanovulation and/or polycystic ovaries, and (3) Exclusion of all other androgen excess or related disorders, which include 21-hydroxylase deficiency, nonclassic adrenal hyperplasia, thyroid dysfunction, hyperprolactinemia, neoplastic androgen secretion, drug-induced androgen excess, syndromes of severe insulin resistance, Cushing's syndrome, and glucocorticoid resistance.

CASE A

Mrs S, a 20-year-old girl, came to our outpatient department (OPD) with complaints of progressive hirsutism, acne, weight gain, and irregular periods for 6 years. She attained menarche at the age of 14 years. The periods were irregular from menarche with a cycle of 20–60 days and the flow of 3–4 days. She had become amenorrheic for the last 6 months, but a recently done progesterone challenge test was positive. Excessive coarse hair growth developed on her chin, upper lips, chest, abdomen, and thighs and progressively increased in the last 2 years. The hair growth is progressively increasing and she has to wax her face once in 10 days. Acne over the face started 2 years back. She has gained 30 kg weight in the last 3 years. She does not control her diet and is fond of eating food with a high fat and carbohydrate content. She has excessive scalp hair loss and frontal balding. Her parents told us that she is depressed and cries often and is very irritable. There was no history of snoring, irregular sleep, or nocturia.

A family history of hirsutism and irregular periods is positive in her mother, who is also obese, weighs 80 kg, and is a type 2 diabetic patient.

On examination, her pulse rate was 78 beats/min, blood pressure (BP) was 140/80 mm Hg, weight was 75 kg, height was 150 cm, and body mass index (BMI) was 33.3 kg/m². She had acanthosis nigricans, skin tags on her neck and axillae, acne on her face and frontal balding, positive abdominal obesity, and white straie over her abdomen. Breasts were stage 5 and there was no galactorrhea, pubic hair stage 5, clitoromegaly was absent, and thyroid was just palpable. She had severe hirsutism with a Ferriman–Gallwey score of 20/36. Her systemic examination was within normal limits.

Investigations

- Thyroid-stimulating hormone (TSH) = 3.3 µU/mL (0.4–4 µU/mL) and free thyroxine (FT4) = 1.19 ng/dL (0.9–2.3 ng/dL)
- Luteinizing hormone (LH) = 11.6 mIU/mL (1.42–15.4 mIU/mL), follicle-stimulating hormone (FSH) = 5.31 mIU/mL (4.7–21 mIU/mL), and prolactin = 12.3 ng/mL (2–25 ng/mL)
- Testosterone = 3.71 ng/mL (<2 ng/mL) and estradiol = 80 pg/mL (30–400 pg/mL)
- Dehydroepiandrosterone sulfate (DHEAS) = 177.3 µg/dL (65–180 µg/dL) and anti-Müllerian hormone (AMH) = 4 ng/mL (0.7–1.0 ng/mL)
- Serum cortisol 8 AM = 11.99 µg/dL (5–23 µg/dL)
- 17-alpha-hydroxyprogesterone 1 hour after synacthen 250 µg intravenous (IV) stat = 2 ng/mL [>10 ng/mL is diagnostic of late-onset congenital adrenal hyperplasia (CAH)]
- Oral glucose tolerance test (OGTT) with 75 g glucose at 0 hour = 88 mg/dL and at 2 hours = 220 mg/dL
- Lipid profile
- Serum cholesterol = 300 mg/dL
- Serum low-density lipoprotein (LDL) = 160 mg/dL
- Serum triglycerides = 250 mg/dL
- Ultrasound of the pelvis
- Both ovaries are bulky, right ovary = 14 mL and left ovary = 16 mL with increased stroma. The right ovary has 12 follicles arranged in the periphery. The left ovary has 15 follicles arranged in the periphery

DIFFERENTIAL DIAGNOSIS

Secondary amenorrhea is defined as no menstruation for more than three cycles, if previously cycles were regular, or more than six cycles in previously irregular cycles in women with established menses. There are four major causes of secondary amenorrhea: (1) Polycystic ovary syndrome, (2) Hypothalamic amenorrhea, (3) Hyperprolactinemia, and (4) Ovarian failure.

Our patient has irregular periods from menarche and 6 months of secondary amenorrhea. Her progesterone withdrawal test was positive. She has significant hirsutism with a Ferriman–Gallwey score of 16/36, acne and frontal balding are positive, and clitoromegaly is negative. She is obese with a BMI of 33 kg/m². Thus, she has all the clinical features of PCOS. The biochemical evidence of increased serum total testosterone increased AMH levels and LH/FSH ratio of 2 suggests PCOS. Radiological evidence of all the ultrasonography features of PCOS such as the volume of ovaries >10 cc, increased stroma, and >10 peripheral follicles is also present. She does not have galactorrhea and serum prolactin is normal, ruling out hyperprolactinemia. Her thyroid functions are normal. Hypothalamic amenorrhea is ruled out by obesity, absence of a history of stress, and normal gonadotropin and estradiol levels. The normal gonadotropin and estradiol levels also rule out primary ovarian failure. The other causes of androgen excess are late-onset CAH, which normal 17-alpha-hydroxyprogesterone levels after adrenocorticotropic hormone (ACTH) stimulation rules out, absence of ultrasonographic evidence, and only mildly elevated serum total testosterone rules out ovarian neoplasms. Normal DHEAS levels ruled out adrenal neoplasms. The patient did not have any history of steroid intake and the cortisol levels were normal, ruling out exogenous steroid intake and glucocorticoid resistance. Thus, a diagnosis of the PCOS was established. Her glucose tolerance test proved that she has diabetes and she also has dyslipidemia in the form of high cholesterol and triglycerides. The history of irritability, mood swings, depressed mood, and weeping spells indicates significant depression.

DIAGNOSIS

- Polycystic ovarian disease
- Type 2 diabetes mellitus (T2DM)
- Dyslipidemia
- Depression

MANAGEMENT OF THE CASE

Our patient was 20-year-old and unmarried and the problems we wanted to resolve were irregular periods, T2DM, obesity, depression, and hirsutism.

Lifestyle management was started by diet counseling and giving the patient a 1,500 calories low-fat diabetic diet, which was 500 calories lower than the patient's usual diet. She was fond of swimming, so her parents were asked to find a nearby swimming pool membership for her and she was started on 45 minutes swimming daily for 6 days per week.

Psychological counseling and fluoxetine 40 mg daily, an antidepressant that is nonsedating and does not cause weight gain, was started by her psychiatrist.

She was given metformin in a dose of 1 g daily initially, which was increased to 2 g along with a combination of cyproterone acetate and ethinyl estradiol daily for 21 days every month. She was also started on 20 mg of rosuvastatin daily at night.

She responded well to her treatment and followed a regular diet and exercise schedule. She was much more confident and had lost 3 kg weight after 3 months of treatment. Her periods were now regular with a cycle of 30 days and 4 days bleeding. Her main problem now was hirsutism, for which she was given laser therapy, six sittings in 2 months. Laser therapy proved effective and her self-esteem improved further.

After a year, she had lost 10 kg weight, was not depressed anymore, frontal balding had improved, hirsutism was controlled, and her blood sugars and lipid levels were under control.

She is on a 3-monthly follow-up schedule with an endocrinologist, nutritionist, and psychiatrist.

DISCUSSION AND REVIEW OF LITERATURE

Hyperinsulinemia and insulin resistance are the critical factors for hyper-androgenism, probably due to the amplification of tropic hormones on steroidogenesis. The role and beneficial effects of insulin sensitizers such as metformin and thiazolidinediones also support this concept of the pathogenic role of insulin resistance as the central and critical pathogenic mechanism of this disorder. Insulin resistance is a pathophysiological contributor in around 50–80% of women with PCOS, particularly in those with more severe PCOS diagnosed based on the NIH criteria in overweight women. Obesity in PCOS patients appears to have a deleterious synergistic effect on glucose homeostasis and predisposing to increase risk of development of frank T2DM.

Although many metabolic disorders can occur in PCOS subjects, the degree of expression is highly variable among individuals. Among the metabolic manifestations, obesity, hyperlipidemia, hyperinsulin-emia, insulin resistance, beta-cell dysfunction, and T2DM are prevalent in addition to increased risk of cardiovascular disease and proposed endometrial cancer. In several studies, autoimmune role in pathophysiologic mechanism is also suggested. The role of genetic susceptibility is also suggested in the literature and familial clustering is found in female relatives of affected patients.

In PCOS, hyperinsulinemia augments androgen production by directly stimulating LH activity through stimulation of ovarian receptors of insulin or insulin-like growth factors or indirectly increasing the amplitude of serum LH pulses. Hyperinsulinemia also decreases serum sex hormone-binding globulin (SHBG) levels and increases free testosterone levels available to act on target organs.

Luteinizing hormone hypersecretion increases serum immunoreactive and bioactive LH levels in about 70% of women with PCOS. Increased LH pulse frequency in PCOS from enhanced hypothalamic gonadotropin-releasing hormone (GnRH) pulsatile release occurs owing to reduced steroid hormone negative feedback on LH secretion because of androgen excess. This neuroendocrine abnormality occurs in adolescent girls with PCOS.

Women with PCOS have a genetic basis triggered by an environmental insult. The first, a locus on chromosome 19p is associated with high susceptibility to PCOS. The second is the fat mass and obesity-associated gene, whose polymorphism has been associated with PCOS. Genome-wide association studies (GWAS) have provided insight into the genetic architecture of PCOS. Studies have evaluated the role of several of the newly identified PCOS risk loci including luteinizing hormone/choriogonadotropin receptor (LHCGR), thyroid adenoma associated (THADA) protein, and differentially expressed in normal and neoplastic cells domain-containing 1A (DENND1A) protein in the pathophysiology of PCOS.

Polycystic ovary syndrome is present in up to 30% of women presenting with secondary amenorrhea. Hyperandrogenemia is present in 60–80% of women, i.e., increased testosterone and DHEAS. Free testosterone assays have been found to be inaccurate and have many variabilities. Assessment of free androgen index will be more useful (100 × total testosterone/SHBG) in PCOS. Serum prolactin levels are elevated in 10–25% of women with PCOS. The LH/FSH ratio is usually >2. About 4% of women with amenorrhea may have abnormal thyroid function. One-fifth of women with regular cycles have ovaries that are polycystic and hyperandrogenic women with PCOS may have regular menstrual cycles.

A study among 105 premenopausal north Indian women with T2DM regarding the prevalence of ultrasonography proved polycystic ovaries 60.95% were documented to have polycystic ovaries compared to 36.66% of the nondiabetic control, which is much higher than the reported prevalence among the normal female population. No significant difference was found regarding PCOS prevalence among obese and nonobese women with T2DM. Diabetic patients with PCOS had significantly higher mean LH, total testosterone, and androstenedione than diabetic females without PCOS.

In a study among 168 young women who attended the endocrine clinic in AIIMS for hirsutism and/or oligomenorrhea, the incidence of glucose intolerance was found in 41.6% of subjects while applying the World Health Organization (WHO) 1999 criteria. Among these, 8.93% had DM, 29.16% had impaired glucose tolerance (IGT), and 3.57% had impaired fasting glucose

(IFG). This estimated prevalence is much higher than otherwise normal women of reproductive age group shown by earlier studies. While applying the 1999 American Diabetes Association (ADA) criteria, only 3.5% of PCOS women had DM and 8.91% had IFG. Significant insulin resistance (44.7%) was found in both obese and nonobese PCOS groups of which 15.47% had severe insulin resistance. Positive family history of known diabetes was present in 47.2% of PCOS females, 26.19% had a family history of hirsutism, and 24.4% had menstrual abnormalities, concluding that Indian women with PCOS have a very high prevalence of glucose intolerance, DM, and insulin resistance and the constellation starts at an early age. A study regarding the prevalence of metabolic syndrome in the family members of women with PCOS from north India revealed first-degree relatives of women with PCOS had a higher presence of metabolic syndrome indicating that they are at a higher risk category for the disorder. Maximum subjects of both PCOS women and their relatives had dyslipidemia, low high-density lipoprotein (HDL), and high triglyceride levels. Serum fasting insulin levels were elevated in index patients and their family members. Insulin sensitivity indices were comparable between groups, indicated high insulin resistance in the families, which might be a heritable trait indicating the need for further molecular genetics studies.

Various treatment approaches to decrease androgen production are ovarian wedge resection, ovarian drilling, luteinizing hormone-releasing hormone (LHRH) analogs, aromatase inhibitors, antiandrogens, and oral contraceptive pills (OCPs). For many years, the OCPs have been the core therapy for PCOS. The combined oral contraceptives (COCs) are those more frequently used for this purpose.

Flutamide is a nonsteroidal selective androgen receptor inhibitor, inhibits the 5-alpha reductase enzyme, which converts testosterone to dihydrotestosterone in target tissues. Flutamide reduces the clinical and biochemical androgenic manifestations and reduces total cholesterol, LDL cholesterol, and triglycerides in women with PCOS.

Spironolactone has been used as an antiandrogen and acts as a steroid synthesis inhibitor. It has been used mainly as a treatment of hirsutism, besides use as a diuretic. Management of PCOS with insulin sensitizers such as thiazolidinedione and metformin that target the dominant pathogenic factor of insulin resistance has gained an area of interest. Metformin also has an insulin-independent mechanism by directly inhibiting theca cell androgen synthesis. Studies have previously reported comparable efficacy of low-dose spironolactone to that of metformin in the management of PCOS.

In a 6-month open-labeled study comparing the efficacy of low-dose spironolactone in combination with metformin, the critical finding suggested superiority of efficacy of the combination of low-dose spironolactone over either drug alone in the management of PCOS without increasing the adverse event rate and did not induce any menstrual irregularities to affect patient compliance.

OVARIAN HYPERTHECOSIS

Ovarian hyperthecosis is a severe variant of PCOS. There is markedly increased androgen production leading to virilization with severe hirsutism and clitoromegaly. The serum testosterone may exceed 2 ng/mL. There is significantly increased stromal tissue with luteinized theca-like cells scattered throughout large sheets of fibroblast-like cells. Treatment of hyperthecosis is difficult and even GnRH analogs cannot suppress testosterone secretion and bilateral oophorectomy is sometimes necessary. Induction of ovulation in these women is difficult, as they do not respond to clomiphene citrate or recombinant FSH.

CONCLUSION

The Androgen Excess Society definition of PCOS is practical and has laid to rest many controversies.

The management of the woman with PCOS depends on her priorities. If she wants children then induction of ovulation, lifestyle changes and metformin therapy is the choice of therapy. If relief of hirsutism and cosmetic improvement is her first priority then lifestyle changes, oral contraceptives with spironolactone and laser therapy is the choice of therapy. Concomitant glucose intolerance and T2DM is treated with metformin therapy. Depression and dyslipidemia have also to be taken care off. It has to be made clear to the patient that PCOS is a chronic disease and the treatment will continue for her entire life.

SUGGESTED READINGS

1. Abbot DH, Dumesic DA, Franks S. Developmental origin of polycystic ovary syndrome—a hypothesis. J Clin Endocrinol. 2002;174:1-5.
2. Adams J, Polson DW, and Franks S. Prevalence of polycystic ovaries in women with anovulation and idiopathic hirsutism. BMJ. 1986;293:355-9.
3. Azziz R, Carmina E, Dewailly D, Kandarakis ED, Morreale HFE, Futterweit W, et al. Position statement: criteria for defining polycystic ovary syndrome as a predominantly hyperandrogenic syndrome: an Androgen Excess Society guideline. J Clin Endocrinol Metab. 2006;91:4237-45.
4. Bergh C, Carlsson B, Olsson JH, Selleskog U, Hillensjo T. Regulation of androgen production in cultured human thecal cells by insulin-like growth factor 1 and insulin. Fertil Steril. 1993;59:323-31.
5. Brown J, Farquhar C, Lee O, Toomath R, Jepson RG. Spironolactone versus placebo or in combination with steroids for hirsutism and/or acne. Cochrane Database Syst Rev. 2009;2:CD000194.
6. Carney AH, Chan KL, Short F, White D, Williamson R, Franks S. Evidence for a single gene effect causing polycystic ovaries and male pattern baldness. Clin Endocrinol (Oxf). 1993;38:653-8.
7. Comim FV, Teerds K, Hardy K, Franks S. Increased protein expression of LHCG receptor and 17-alpha-hydroxylase/17-20-lyase in human polycystic ovaries. Hum Reprod. 2013;28:3086-92.
8. Corvol P, Michaud A, Menard J, Friefeld M, Mahoudean J. Antiandrogenic effect of spironolactone: mechanism of action. Endocrinology. 1975;97:52-8.
9. Diamanti-Kandarakis E, Mitrakou A, Raptis S, Tolis G, Duleba AJ. The effect of a pure antiandrogen receptor blocker, flutamide, on the lipid profile in the polycystic ovary syndrome. J Clin Endocrinol Metab. 1998;83:2699-705.

10. Dunaif A, Graf M, Mendeli J, Laumas U, Dobrjansky A. Characterization of groups of hyperandrogenic women with acanthosis nigricans, impaired glucose tolerance and/or hyperinsulinemia. J Clin Endocrinol. 1987;65:499-507.

11. Dunaif A. Insulin resistance and the polycystic ovary syndrome: mechanism and implications for pathogenesis. Endocrine Rev. 1997;18:774-800.

12. Escobar-Morreale HF. Polycystic ovary syndrome: treatment strategies and management. Exp Opin Pharmacother. 2008;9:2995-3008.

13. Franks S. Polycystic ovary syndrome. N Engl J Med. 1995;333:853-61.

14. Ganie MA, Khurana ML, Eunice M, Gupta N, Dwivedi SN, Gulati SN, et al. Prevalence of glucose intolerance among adolescent and young women with polycystic ovary syndrome in India. Indian J Endocrinol Metab. 2004;6:9-14.

15. Ganie MA, Khurana ML, Eunice M, Gupta N, Gulati M, Dwivedi SN, et al. Comparison of efficacy of spironolactone with metformin in the management of polycystic ovary syndrome: an open-labeled study. J Clin Endocrinol Metab. 2004;89:2756-62.

16. Ganie MA, Khurana ML, Nisar S, Shah PA, Shah ZA, Kulshrestha B, et al. Improved efficacy of low-dose spironolactone and metformin combination than either drug alone in the management of women with polycystic ovary syndrome (PCOS): a six-month, open-label randomized study. J Clin Endocrinol Metab. 2013;98:3599-607.

17. Ganie MA, Marwaha RK, Aggarwal R, Singh S. High prevalence of polycystic ovary syndrome characteristics in girls with euthyroid chronic lymphocytic thyroiditis. A case-control study. Eur J Endocrinol. 2010;162:1-7.

18. Goyal A, Malhotra R, Kulshrestha V, Kachhawa G. Severe hyperandrogenism due to ovarian hyperthecosis in a young woman. BMJ Case Rep. 2019;12:e232783.

19. Knochenhauer ES, Key TJ, Kahsar-Miller M, Waggoner W, Boots LR, Aziz R. Prevalence of the polycystic ovary syndrome in unselected black and white women of the southeastern United States: a prospective study. J Clin Endocrinol Metab. 1998;83:3078-82.

20. Legro RS, Driscoll D, Strauss JF, Fox J, Dunaif A. Evidence for a genetic basis for hyper-androgenemia in polycystic ovary syndrome. Proc Natl Acad Sci U S A. 1998;95:14956-60.

21. Lobo RA, Shoupe D, Serafini P, Brinton D, Horton R. The effects of two doses of spironolactone on serum androgens and anagen hair in hirsute women. Fertil Steril. 1985;43:200-5.

22. McAllister JM, Modi B, Miller BA, Biegler J, Bruggeman R, Legro RS, et al. Overexpression of a DENND1A isoform produces a polycystic ovary syndrome theca phenotype. Proc Natl Acad Sci U S A. 2014;111:1519-27.

23. Rotterdam ESHRE/ASRM-Sponsored PCOS Consensus Workshop Group. Revised 2003 consensus on diagnostic criteria and long-term health risks related to polycystic ovary syndrome. Fertil Steril. 2004;81:19-25.

24. Sattar N, Hopkinson ZOC, Green IA. Insulin sensitizing agents in polycystic ovary syndrome. Lancet. 1998;351:305-7.

25. Shabir I, Ganie MA, Zargar MA, Bhat D, Mir MM, Jan A, et al. Prevalence of metabolic syndrome in the family members of women with polycystic ovary syndrome from north India. Indian J Endocrinol Metab. 2014;18:364-9.

26. Spritzer PM, Lisboa KO, Mattiello S, Lhullier F. Spironolactone as a single agent for long-term therapy of hirsute patients. Clin Endocrinol (Oxf). 2000;52:587-94.

27. Tsilchorozidou T, Overton C, Conway GS. The pathophysiology of polycystic ovary syndrome. Clin Endocrinol (Oxf). 2004;60:1-17.

28. Viollet B, Guigas B, Sanz-Garcia N, Leclerc J, Foretz M, Andreelli F. Cellular and molecular mechanisms of metformin: an overview. Clin Sci (Lond). 2012;122:253-70.

29. Wang P, Zhao H, Li T, Zhang W, Wu K, Li M, et al. Hypomethylation of the LH/choriogonadotropin receptor promoter region is a potential mechanism underlying susceptibility to polycystic ovary syndrome. Endocrinology. 2014;155:1445-52.

30. Zargar AH, Gupta VK, Wani AI, Masoodi SR, Bashir MI, Laway BA, et al. Prevalence of ultrasonography proved polycystic ovaries in North Indian women with type 2 diabetes mellitus. Reprod Biol Endocrinol. 2005;3:35.

31. Zawadzki JK, Dunaif A. Diagnostic criteria for polycystic ovary syndrome: towards a rational approach. In: Zawadzki JK, Dunaif A (Eds). Current Issues in Endocrinology and Metabolism. Boston: Blackwell Scientific; 1992. pp. 377-84.

INDEX

Page numbers followed by *b* refer to box, *f* refer to figure, *fc* refer to flowchart, and *t* refer to table